Advances in Hematologic Malignancies

Edited by Gamal Abdul Hamid

Published in London, United Kingdom

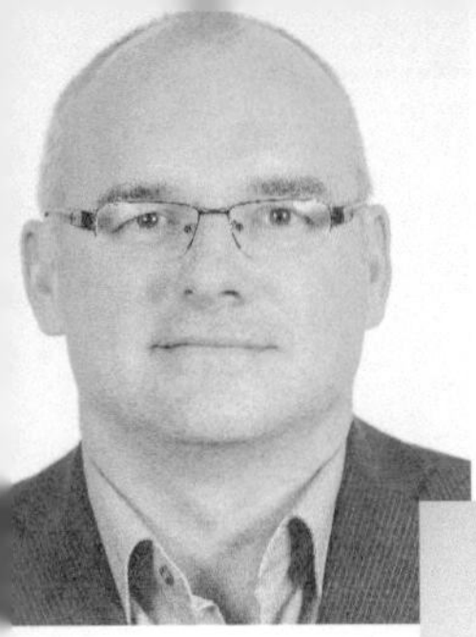
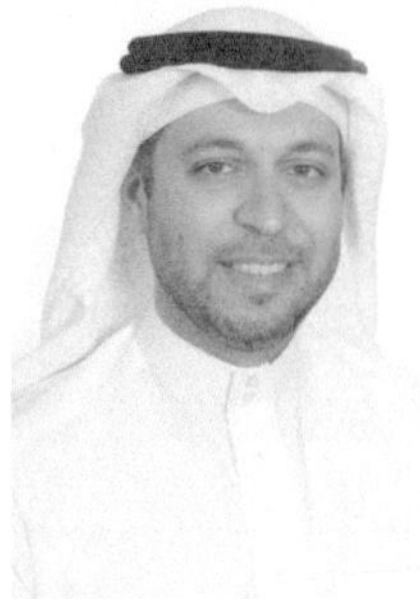
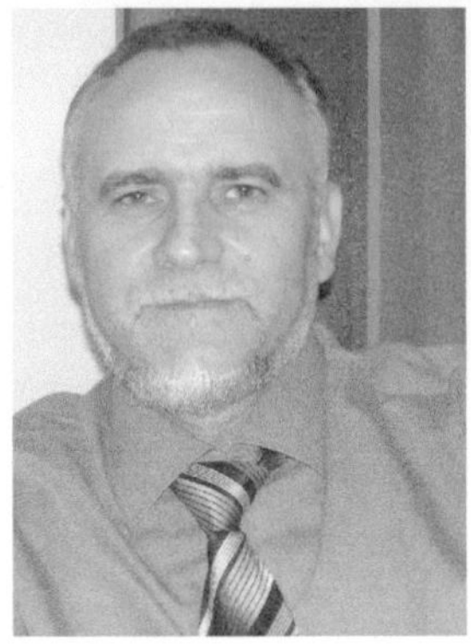
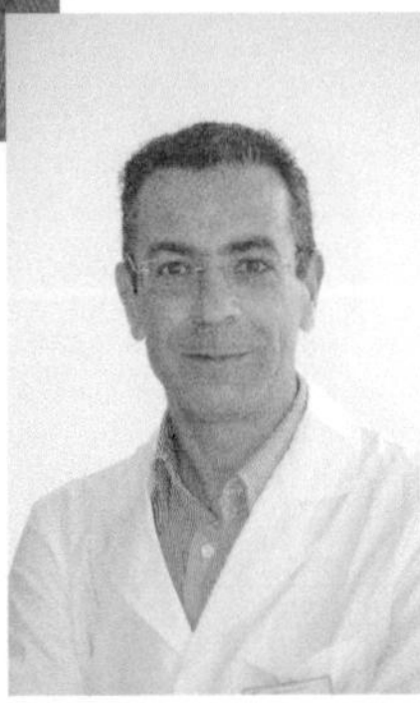
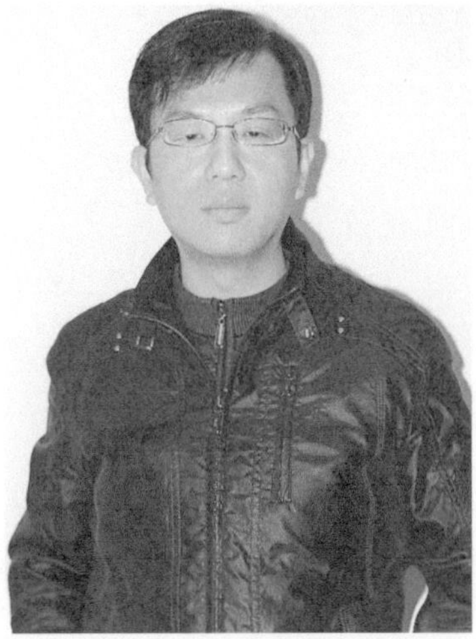
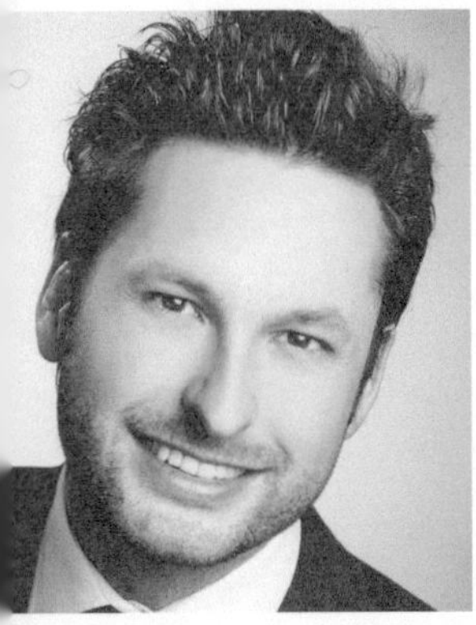
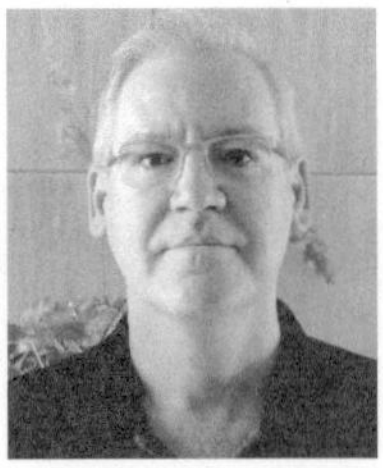

IntechOpen

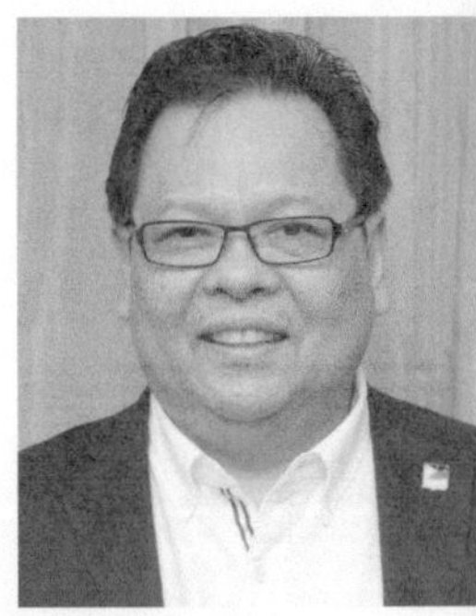
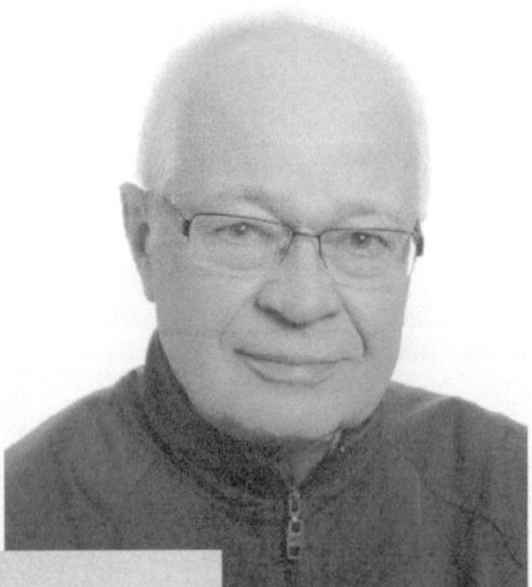
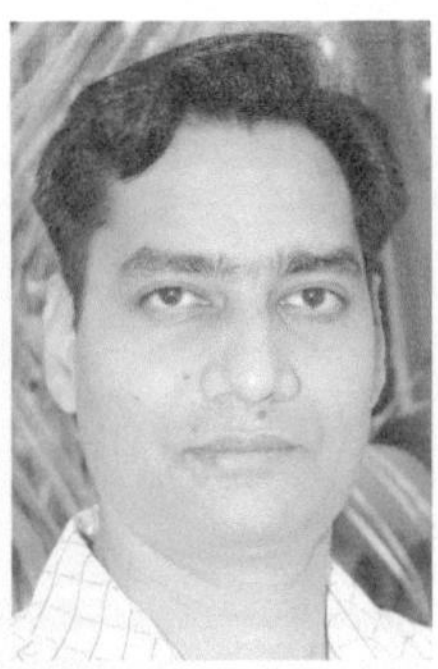
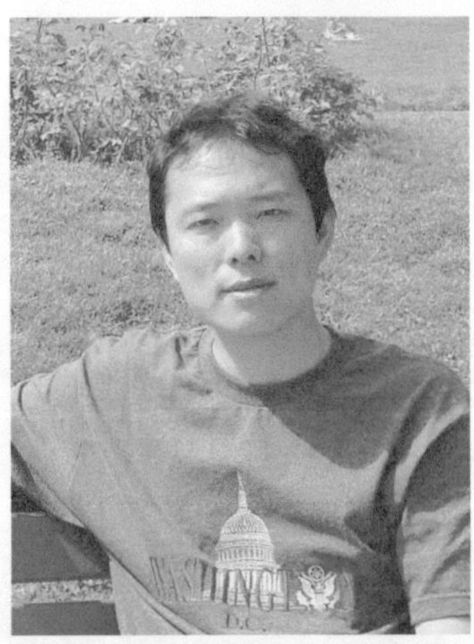
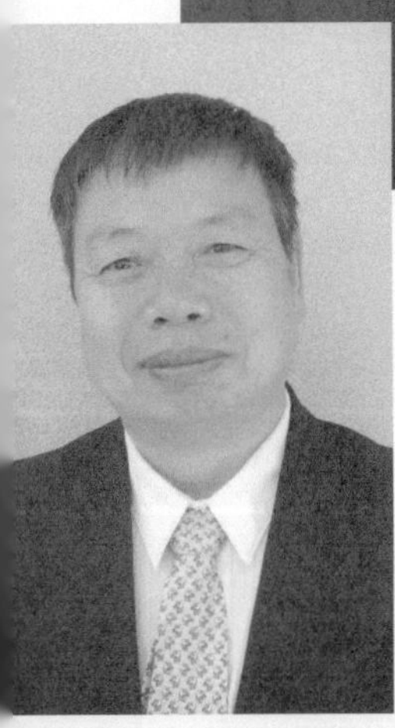
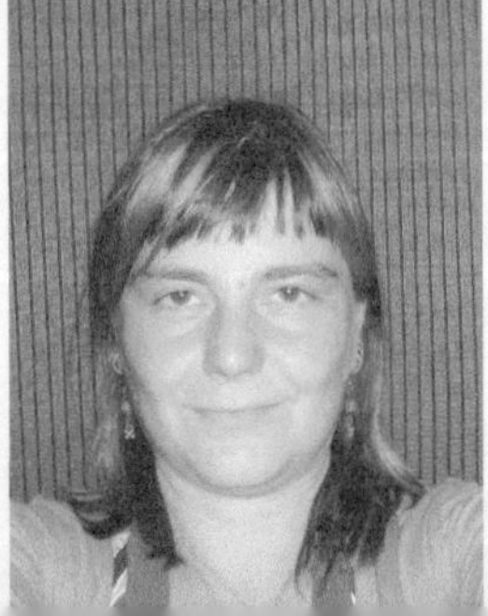

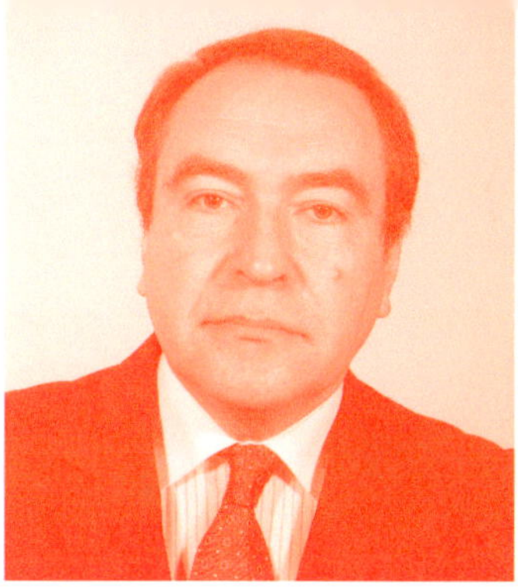
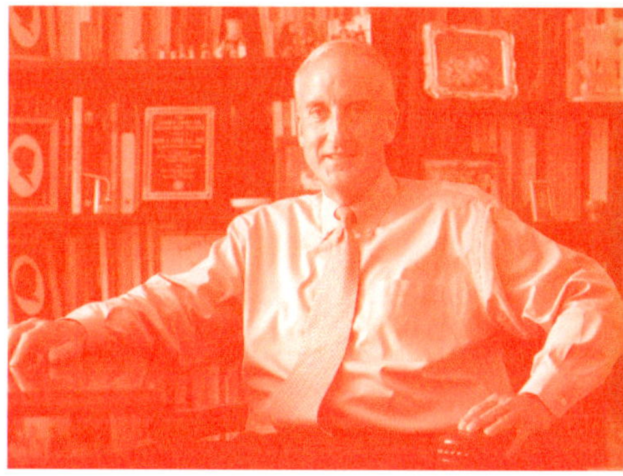
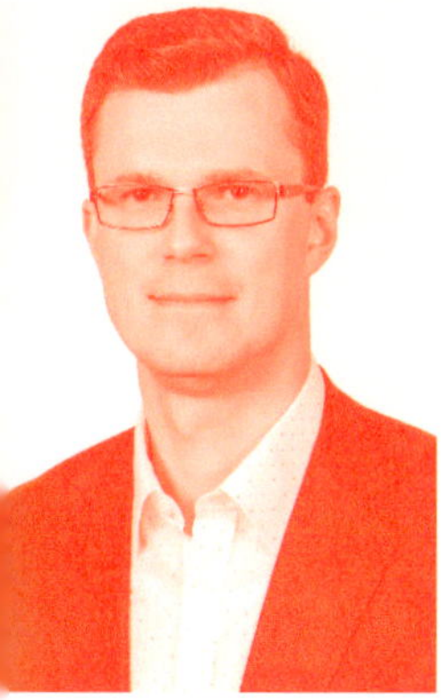
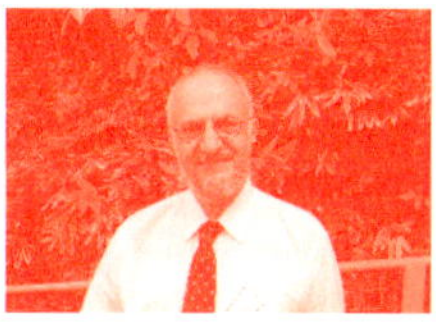
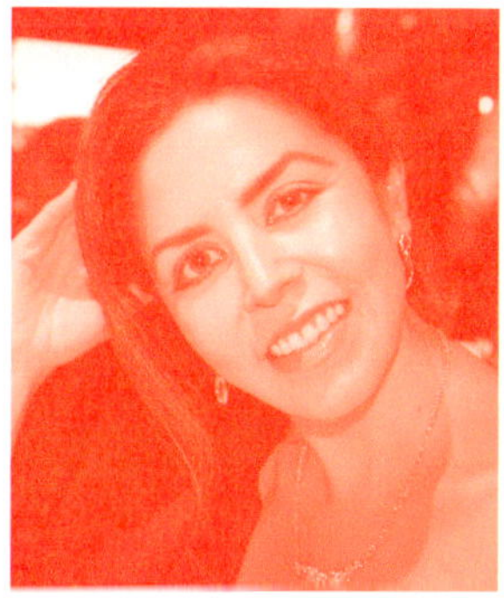

Supporting open minds since 2005

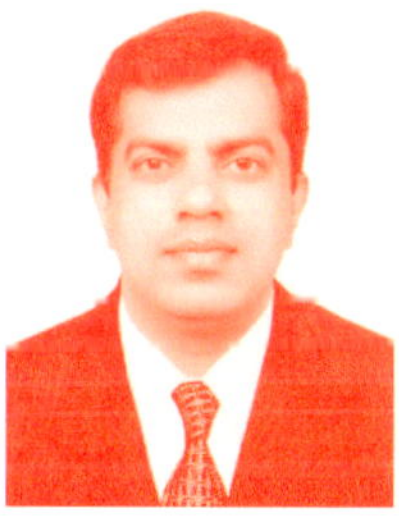
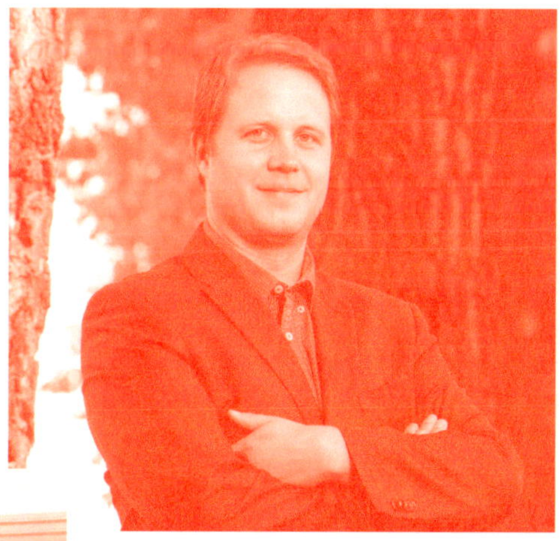
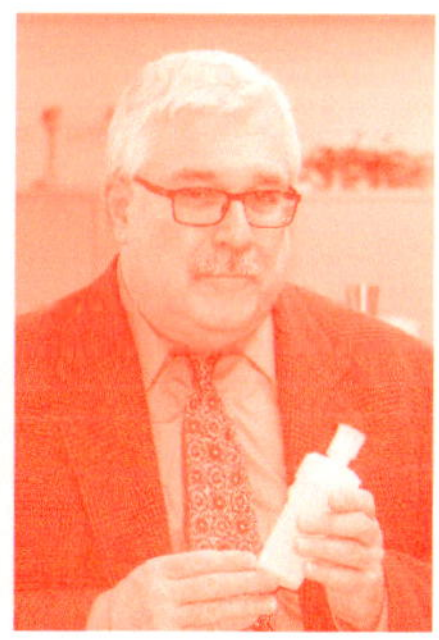
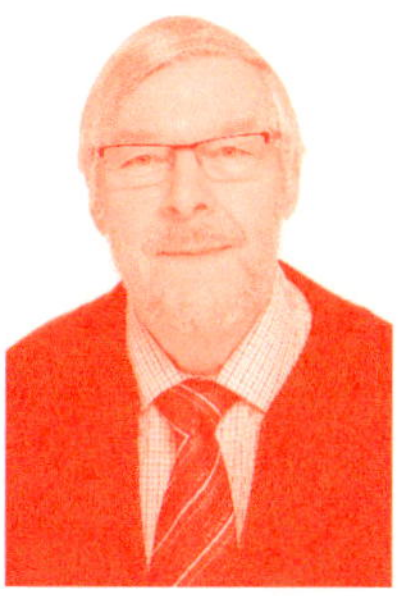
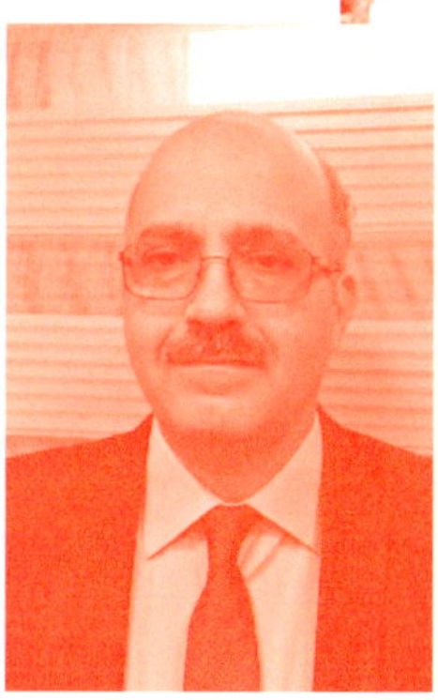
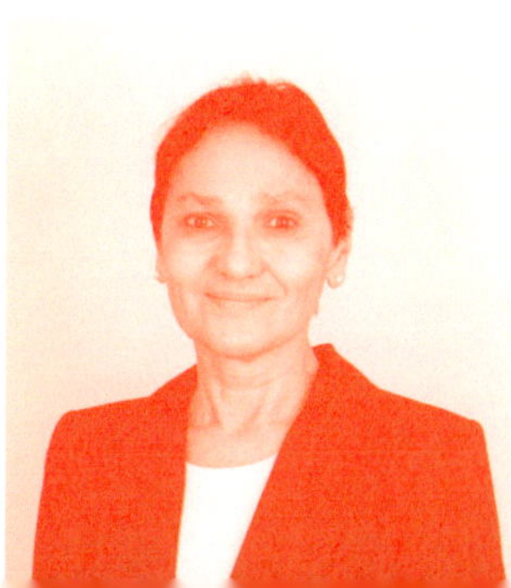
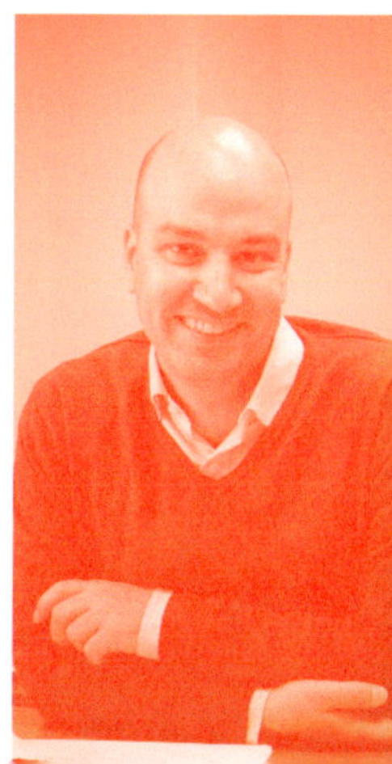

Advances in Hematologic Malignancies
http://dx.doi.org/10.5772/intechopen.77785
Edited by Gamal Abdul Hamid

Contributors
Haitao Zhu, Xiaoxiao Yang, Xuewen Xu, Yanfang Liu, Aihua Gong, Dongqing Wang, Xiang Liao, Safa Shukry, Abdulwahab Al-Nehmi, Cyrus Khan, Yazan Samhouri, Rupin Shah, Jorge Organista-Nava, Yazmín Gómez-Gómez, Berenice Illades-Aguiar, Marco Antonio Leyva-Vázquez, Gamal Abdul Hamid, Fadhel Hariri, Sneha Tandon, Angela Punnett, Tomas Dobransky, Martina Madarova, Dominik Dobransky, Amit Garg, Tarveen Jandoo, Deepak Csn, Omar Aljitawi

First published in London, United Kingdom, 2019 by IntechOpen
IntechOpen is the global imprint of INTECHOPEN LIMITED, registered in England and Wales, registration number: 11086078, 7th floor, 10 Lower Thames Street, London, EC3R 6AF, United Kingdom
Printed in Croatia

British Library Cataloguing-in-Publication Data
A catalogue record for this book is available from the British Library

Additional hard and PDF copies can be obtained from orders@intechopen.com

Advances in Hematologic Malignancies
Edited by Gamal Abdul Hamid
p. cm.
Print ISBN 978-1-78923-941-6
Online ISBN 978-1-78923-942-3
eBook (PDF) ISBN 978-1-83962-657-9

For EU product safety concerns:
IN TECH d.o.o., Prolaz Marije Krucifikse Kozulić 3, 51000 Rijeka, Croatia, info@intechopen.com or visit our website at intechopen.com.

Meet the editor

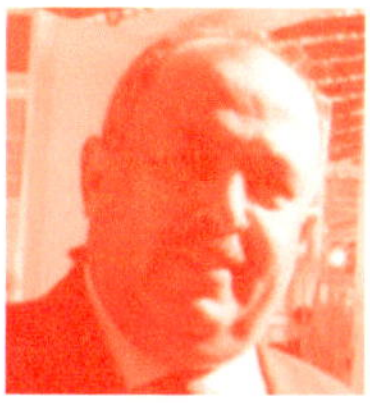

Prof Dr Gamal Abdul Hamid received his German Board certification in internal medicine and his PhD in hematology-oncology from the Faculty of Medicine (Caral Gustav Carus), University of Dresden from 1987 to 1993. Currently, he is working as the Director of the National Program of Cancer Control in Yemen and he is the head of hematology and clinical laboratory in the Faculty of Medicine, University of Aden. He is the General Secretary of the Yemen Cancer Society and founder of Aden Cancer Registry. He is serving as an editorial member of several journals, has authored or co-authored many articles in a great variety of journals and has delivered lectures at many conferences and institutions in Yemen and internationally and has also reviewed national and international journals. He is a member of European Society for Medical Oncology (ESMO), American Society of Clinical Oncology (ASCO), International Network For Cancer Treatment and Research (INCTR), and Pan Arab Oncology.

Contents

Preface

This book presents the advances, progress and current knowledge on hematologic malignancies.

Advances in Hematologic Malignancies contains 9 interesting chapters, each a separate publication that reflects each author's concept and view and concentrates on recent research on molecular pathology, genomic changes, cellular disease processes, and advances in target therapy of hematologic malignancies. There are currently numerous therapeutic options accessible to the modern hematologist and, fortunately, an extraordinarily improved viewpoint for the vast majority of patients with hematological malignancies.

The work presented in this book will be of benefit and a relevant source of knowledge for hematologists, oncologists, pathologists, researcher,s and postgraduate students in hemato-oncology. This book is written by experienced clinicians and researchers from China, Mexico, Canada,USA, Yemen, India, and Brazil.

The editor is thankful for excellent cooperation and support and regular follow up given by Ms Kristina Kardum from IntechOpen.

Gamal Abdul Hamid
Aden University Faculty of Medicine,
Aden, Yemen

Chapter 1

Introductory Chapter: Advances in Hematologic Malignancies

Gamal Abdul Hamid and Fadhel Hariri

1. Introduction

Hematological malignancies contain an accumulation of heterogeneous conditions, by which is commonly affect old ages, as the median age for most of these diseases all originating from cells of the bone marrow and the lymphatic system. There are three noteworthy gatherings: lymphomas, leukemia and plasma cell neoplasms. European patients with hematological malignancies have improved over the previous decade, most likely as a result of new medications, for example, imatinib in chronic myeloid leukemia and rituximab in lymphomas [1].

In developed countries and developing countries hematological malignancies (HMs) are differs and account about 8–9% of all cancers, being the fourth common cancer in developed countries [2]. The leukemia incidence rates are 24.5 per 100,000 is 8.8% in the US, 6.3% in Jordan, 5.4% in Egypt [3] The lymphoma incidence rate have been reported to be high in Canada (27.7%), Australia (25%) and Western Europe (17.9%), moderate (10.2%) in Middle East and Africa and low (6.5%) in East Asia [3].

While the previous 20 years witnessed an explosion in the quantity approved treatments for lymphoid and myeloid malignancies and few medications were endorsed, especially for leukemia, lymphoma and myeloma. This was astounding in light of comparable, if not more prominent, propels in the comprehension of the genetic basis and pathophysiology of hematological malignancies, which account 8–24% of every single grown-up disease [1]. The test of making an interpretation of these logical revelations into powerful treatments for patients with hematological malignancies established as an urgent unmet medical need.

2. Molecular diagnosis in hematological malignancies

Hematological malignancies are heterogeneous in both clinical and biological aspects. The association of genomic profile changes associated with hematological malignancies is complex and variable including translocations, karyotypic improvements, transformations and adjustments of post-translational alteration and some genetic changes are needed, to induce the onset of disease. This proof in relationship with the development of molecular techniques has prompted an alteration of the current authoritative opinion concentrating on a solitary quality or single pathway analysis [4].

The advancement in molecular biology techniques has not just permitted the individualized molecular diagnosis of hematological malignancies but have also prompted the disclosure of genetic or targeted therapeutic schemes with cytotoxic, anti-metabolic or immunomodulatory properties [4].

Utilizing karyotype analysis and the new technique of polymerase chain reaction (PCR), chromosomal microarrays (CMA), fluorescence in situ hybridization (FISH)

IntechOpen

and new generation sequencing technique (NGS), it is conceivable to configuration better hazard stratification classes and decide if there is complete remission or presence of minimal residual disease (MRD).

New molecular and cytogenetic methods have been connected to determination of diagnosis and treatment. As to, the reasonableness of those strategies expands the precision and the speed of results while screening can be even more successfully performed. In regard to treatments, immunomodulatory and target therapies assurance better outcomes with less hematological side effects.

The molecular basis of hematological malignancies has developed aberrant genes expression and/or pathological expression of natural genes [5]. Also other new somatic mutations detected by Next Generation Sequencing NGS have prompted the revelation of already unknown molecular and pathological genes as well as diagnostic and therapeutic value [6].

Genetic changes plays a vital role to diagnose and classify the stage of disease and determine the prognosis of diseases and choice of treatment in most hematological malignancies [7–9]. Molecular diagnostic technology in patients with HMs is useful for diagnosis and prognosis and selecting the proper treatment, and to monitor the degree of response to new therapies [5, 8].

The majority of leukemia, specifically predictable by gene expression profiles [9]. Vulnerability tests are being developed through the explicit treatment of targeted therapies such as imatinib in acute lymphoblastic leukemia BCR-ABL positive (ALL) and farnesyltransferase inhibitors in acute myeloblastic leukemia (AML) [10].

Myelodysplastic syndrome (MDS) and acute leukemia (AML and ALL) are intensely influenced by epigenetics [11]. Targeted epigenetic therapies may be particularly attractive as long-term treatment in post remission period, if they could target certain subclones once standard chemotherapy has produced targeted cytoreduction to induce remission of acute leukemia [12]. Personalized targeted therapy have just upset treatment results in some HMs, especially, chronic myeloid leukemia (CML), non-Hodgkin's lymphoma (NHL), multiple myeloma (MM) and acute promyelocytic leukemia (APL) [12, 13].

3. Detection of molecular markers in hematologic malignancies

The molecular markers and genetic studies in hematologic malignancies include: (1) **AML**: FLT3-ITD, CEBPA, RUNX1, NPM1, PML-RARA, *ASXL1*, IDH1, IDH2, DNMT3A, TET2 and BCR-ABL1; (2) **ALL**: IKFZ1, CDKN2A/B, BCR-ABL1, BCR-ABL1-like, NOTCH1, ETV6, and RUNX1; (3) **chronic myeloproliferative** (CMPNs): CAL-R, MPL, JAK2, SRSF2, SETBP1, *TP53*, CSF3R and ASXL1; (4) **CML**: BCR-ABL1; (5) **MDS**: RUNX1, *JAK2*, EZH2, SF3B1, IDH1/2, *N-RAS*, TP53, TET2, *KIT*, SRSF2, and ASXL1; (6) **CLL**: ATM, TP53, BIRC3, del11q, SF3B1 and NOTCH1 mut; (7) **Hodgkin's lymphoma (HL)**: BCL6, SOC1, JUNB, MAP3K14, STAT6, MDM2, JAK2, XPO1, NFKBIE, GNA13, MAFB,IKBA, TNFIP3, BCL3, NFKBIA, PD-L1, PD-L2, and REL6; (8) **B-cell lymphomas**: MYC/BCL2, MYC/BCL2/BLC6, SOX11, CCND1/2, *CCND3* and *TCF3*; (9) **T-cell lymphomas**: TP63, IRF4, DUSP22 and ALK; (10) **Hairy cell leukemia (HCL)**: BRAFV600E, *IGHV4-34*, *MAP2K1*; and (11) **MM**: KRAS, CCND1, CCND2, CCND3, TP53, DI53, NRAS, MAF, FAM46C and BRAF [5, 10, 14–17].

4. Personalized target therapy: Monoclonal antibodies

In the late 1970s, the technology development of monoclonal antibody (MoAb) was possible to produce antibodies targeting specific antigens to the surface of cancer cells. The antibodies target an antigen present at high concentrations on cancer cells and missing or present at low fixations on typical cells. The MoAbs, is given as monotherapy or target therapy with chemotherapy, have excellent outcome in different types of neoplasm's with improve quality of life and survival rate and time. An assortment of components has been proposed that would allow monoclonal antibodies to kill cancer cells, including apoptosis, inhibition of cell growth, cellular cytotoxicity.

The development of molecular and genetic technology play important role in the modernization and modification of the (2016 WHO Edition) for classification of tumors of hematopoietic and lymphoid tissues, is being published by World Health Organization, the aims to provide these data with essential clinical characteristics, morphology and immunophenotyping relevant to targeted and novel therapies against incurable diseases [18].

The targeted and novel therapies currently used in the treatment of hematological malignancies are: (1) Acute myeloblastic leukemia subtypes: lintuzumab, midostaurin, gemtuzumab, ulocuplumab, sorafinib, navitoclax, panobinostat, vorinostat, Dr383-IL3 and lestaurtinib; (2) acute myeloblastic leukemia (promyelocytic type): all trans-retinoic acid gemtuzumab ozogamicin and arsenic trioxide; (3) acute lymphoblastic leukemia: tyrosine kinase inhibitors, rituximab, inotuzumab ozogamicin, nelarabine, blinatumomab, and CAR T-cells; (4) myelodysplastic syndrome: azacitidine, decitabine, and lenalidomide; (5) chronic myeloid leukemia: imatinib, nilotinib, dasatinib and ponatinib; (6) chronic myeloproliferative neoplasms: ruxolitinib; (7) chronic lymphatic leukemia (CLL): rituximab, idelalisib, ibrutinib, venetoclax obinutuzumab, and duvelisib; (8) HL: brentuximabvedotin, nivolumab, rituximab and everolimus; (9) B-cell lymphomas: tositumomab, rituximab, ibritumomab tiuxetan and CAR T-cells; (10) T-cell lymphomas: romidepsin, alemtuzumab, epratuzumab, denileukin and nelarabine; (11) hairy cell leukemia: vemurafenib; and (12) multiple myeloma: bortezomib, carfilzomib, lenalidomide, pomalidomide, daratumumab milatuzumab, and ixazomib [17–26].

The targeted treatments are directed to the cancer cell and do not harm or affect the healthy cell, which is of course a breakthrough in the treatment of hematological malignancies, but is still in the process of research despite the success of the experiments, which have been conducted and targeted therapies exist for many types of cancers, including: Chronic leukemia and lymphoma is used in making there are opportunities for no need for bone marrow transplantation, and targeted therapies have proven to be a great success.

5. Examples of advance treatment in AML

5.1 Enasidenib for *IDH*-mutated AML

Mutations in isocitrate dehydrogenase (IDH) occur in 20% of AML cases and are also found in gliomas and cholangiocarcinomas. Enasidenib was approved in August 2017 by FDA for treatment acute myeloblastic leukemia patients (AML) refractory or relapsed to chemotherapy with presence of IDH2 mutation. IDH2 mutations are relatively common in hematological malignancies, which occur in ~12% of AML patients [27]. The follow up of patients for a period of 6.6 months, 23% of patients experienced a complete remission [28]. The dose of enasidenib is 100 mg once daily and continuously was chosen for the extension stage.

5.2 Gemtuzumab ozogamicin for CD33+ AML

Gemtuzumab ozogamicin (Mylotarg) is an antibody-drug conjugate to treat patients who are more than 60 years old in first relapse AML with CD33+ and not candidates for chemotherapy and also for pediatric patients, more than 2 years old with relapsed or refractory CD33+ AML. Subsequent studies with positive findings resulted in the resurrection of gemtuzumab ozogamicin and its approval in 2017.

5.3 Midostaurin in *FLT3*-mutated AML

Midostaurin was approved on 28 April 2017 by FDA for patients with AML who had FLT3 mutations. Midostaurin is an oral small molecule FLT3 inhibitor that inhibits wild-type and mutant FLT3 kinases as well as a number of other factors. The recommended dose of midostaurin is 50 mg capsules given twice daily on days 8–21, with cytarabine (200 mg/m^2), continuously for 7 days (d1–7) and 60 mg/m^2 daunorubicin for 3 days on (d1–3) and also repeat same dose of midostaurin daily for 2 weeks (day 8–21) in each cycle of consolidation in combination with high dose of cytarabine [29].

6. Some target therapy experience in lymphoproliferative neoplasms

6.1 Rituximab in the treatment of non-Hodgkin's lymphoma

Rituximab (RTX), a chimeric mouse anti-human monoclonal antibodies (MoAbs) targets the CD20 antigen expressed on the neoplastic B cells of leukemia and lymphoma. Rituximab approved by FDA n 1997 for the treatment of B-cell CD20 positive relapsed and refractory of indolent follicular lymphoma, and the European Medicines Agency approved rituximab in June 1998 for chemoresistant or relapsed NHL and for therapy of patients with stage III/IV [7].

The expression of CD20 is varies according to type of cancer (expression in follicular lymphoma is very high, while in chronic lymphocytic leukemia is low). The R-CHOP combination chemotherapy protocol (rituximab, cyclophosphamide, oncovin adriamycin and prednisone) has shown better survival than CHOP alone for treatment of high grade diffuse large cell lymphoma (DLBCL).

6.2 Alemtuzumab for *patients* chronic lymphocytic leukemia

Alemtuzumab is a recombinant humanized immunoglobulin MoAb that targets the cell-surface CD52 antigen, has indicated promising outcomes. CD52 is expressed at high levels on normal healthy cells and on CLL cells. Alemtuzumab initially received FDA-approved in September 2007 for treatment of B-CLL patients who are refractory to chemotherapy (fludarabine-*refractory* CLL) [30].

6.3 Milatuzumab in the treatment of multiple myeloma

Milatuzumab is an anti-CD74 monoclonal antibody express the CD47 antigen.

Anti-CD47 antibodies have emerged in recent years as a new class of checkpoint inhibitors that may be useful target therapy of hematological malignancies and more effective in treatment of MM, CLL and NHL [31]. Milatuzumab in single monotherapy or in combination with bortezomib is very effective in multiple myeloma.

6.4 Epratuzumab

Epratuzumab targets the CD22 antigen on B lymphocytes and has additionally been utilized against refractory or relapsed DLBCL patients to rituximab and can be given as monotherapy or in combination with rituximab or standard chemotherapy achieved complete remission in 60% of patients [32].

6.5 Inotuzumab ozogamicin for Philadelphia+ ALL

Like gemtuzumab ozogamicin, inotuzumab ozogamicin (Besponsa), an antibody/chemotherapy conjugate that internalizes into the tumor cells upon binding to CD22 on the cell surface. "It's carrying a CD22 Trojan horse to the cell, discharging the payload there (the microtubule-targeting agent calicheamicin) is a highly potent chemotherapeutic drug belonging to the enediyne class of DNA-damaging cytotoxic agents derived from the soil bacterium *Micromonospora echinospora* ssp. calichensis." Inotuzumab looks encouraging in a number of lymphomas, yet it came to advertise first for relapsed or refractory B-ALL patients. The pivotal multicenter stage III preliminary selected 326 patients with refractory or relapsed ALL CD22+, randomizing them to a standard treatment or inotuzumab ozogamicin [33]. Its recent approval has greatly increased the ability to attain remission long period and represents a significant advance in therapeutic options for treatment of relapsed ALL.

6.6 Copanlisib for follicular lymphoma

In September, 2017, Copanlisib *was* approved *by the FDA* used to treat of adult patients with recurrent low grade follicular lymphoma who have received at least two previous chemotherapies. Copanlisib is a class I phosphatidylinositol 3-kinase (PI3K) inhibitor with a predominance of PI3K-α and PI3K-δ activity present in cancerous B cells [34].

6.7 Ibrutinib in chronic graft-vs.-host disease (GVHD)

In 2017, ibrutinib (Imbruvica) was approved as the first drug for GVHD after corticosteroid therapies response failure. Ibrutinib is a small-molecule of the B-cell antigen receptor inhibits cell proliferation, and promotes apoptosis of cancer cells through inhibition of Bruton's tyrosine kinase. The daily oral dose of 420 mg with median time response of 12 weeks and overall response rate about 67% [35].

7. CAR T-cell therapy

In fact, the new therapeutic progress of chimeric antigen receptor T cell is simultaneously a genetically, mechanically, and cellular therapy. This technique changed the leukocytes of the patient in such a way that they could identify and destroy the cancer cells. Despite a number of side effects, CAR T-Cell therapy will be effective for most patients who do not accept any other treatment or in relapses.

The purpose of CAR creation is to attack specific target molecules on the surface of cancer cells. They are usually antigens CD19 and CD22, which are designated for malignant cells in leukemia and lymphoma. It is very important that there are no similar molecules on the surface of healthy cells. The patient's own T cells are designed to show antigen receptors as "warheads" to focus on and assault tumor cells tumor cells when infused back into the patient. At the point when T cells perceive their target, they are activated, prompting the release of natural killer cells, cytokines, cytotoxic T lymphocytes, and other effector components.

The test of these engineered cells is to avoid inhibitor and suppressive signals from regulatory immune cells, the target cells, and the tumor microenvironment. It is beneficial to make reference to that CAR-T cell can recognize potential antigens in almost all structures including lipid, carbohydrate and protein antigens, which can be joined explicitly by antibodies [36, 37].

To make a situation where the CAR T cells will be respected, the patient experiences lymphodepleting treatment with fludarabine and cyclophosphamide. A couple of days after the fact, the T-cell item is transfused into the patient, where CD8+ and CD4+ cells will extend and endure until the tumor is dispensed with. Whenever effective, this procedure prompts long-term remission [38, 39].

In August 2017, a number of large clinical trials of the new cancer treatment technique, CAR T-cell, were completed. According to their findings, two drugs were approved by FDA: tisagenlecleucel (Kymriah) and as the first synthetic therapy for relapsed or refractory B- ALL and the second product of CAR T-cell therapy is axicabtagene ciloleucel (Yescarta), as immunotherapy for adults patients whose large cell lymphoma in refractory or relapsed on other therapies, including high-grade large cell lymphoma (mediastinal or transformed from follicular lymphoma) [38].

The improvement method of treatment with of CAR T cell therapy requires experience in many areas, including biology, molecular biology, antibody technology, regulatory requirements, and more. Increasing collaboration among key specialists from universities, research centers, and stakeholders will enhance the success of these drugs [39].

8. Bone marrow transplantation

Bone marrow transplantation is an important branch and important indicator of the treatment model of hematologic malignancies. Hematopoietic stem cell transplantation (HSCT) has been included in therapeutic guidelines for most malignant tumors [40]. For those diseases that can be treated by a conventional therapy, how many of the acute leukemia and aggressive lymphomas and allogeneic BMT they are often the preferred treatment, if the initial relapse. For hematologic malignancies curable with a conventional therapy, such as multiple myeloma, myelodysplastic syndromes and low-grade lymphoma and acute leukemia poor risk, usually the treatment will be allogeneic BMT treatment at the time survival duration is felt to be relatively short.

Author details

Gamal Abdul Hamid[1*] and Fadhel Hariri[2]

1 Faculty of Medicine, Aden University, Aden, Yemen

2 Ministry of Public Health, Aden, Yemen

*Address all correspondence to: drgamal2000@yahoo.com

References

[1] Munro AJ. Leukaemia and lymphoma: Why has survival improved? The Lancet Oncology. 2014;**15**:906-907. DOI: 10.1016/S1470-2045(14)70312-2

[2] Smith A, Howell D, Patmore R. Incidence of haematological malignancy by sub-type: A report from the Haematological Malignancy Research Network. British Journal of Cancer. 2011;**105**(11):1684-1692. DOI: 10.1038/bjc.2011.450

[3] Hamid GA. Pattern of hematological malignancies in Al-Gamhouria Teaching Hospital, Aden, Yemen 2008-2010. Turkish Journal of Hematology. 2012;**29**:342-347. DOI: 10.5505/tjh.2012.0376

[4] Bowman RL, Busque L, Levine RL. Clonal hematopoiesis and evolution to hematopoietic malignancies. Cell Stem Cell. 2018;**22**(2):157-170. DOI: 10.1016/j.stem.2018.01.011

[5] Braggio E, Egan JB, Fonseca R, et al. Lessons from next-generation sequencing analysis in hematological malignancies. Blood Cancer Journal. 2013;**3**:e127. DOI: 10.1038/bcj.2013.26

[6] Prakash G, Kaur A, Malhotra P, et al. Current role of genetics in hematologic malignancies. Indian Journal of Hematology and Blood Transfusion. 2016;**32**(1):18-31. DOI: 10.1007/s12288-015-0584-4. Epub: September 16, 2015

[7] Glennie MJ, French RR, Cragg MS, et al. Mechanisms of killing by anti-CD20 monoclonal antibodies. Molecular Immunology. 2007;**44**:3823-3837. DOI: 10.1016/j.molimm.2007.06.151

[8] Wan TK. Molecular cytogenetics: Techniques, developments and applications. The Journal of Hong Kong Institute of Medical Laboratory Sciences. 2009-2010;**12**(1&2):1-12

[9] Serratì S, De Summa S, Pilato B, et al. Next-generation sequencing: Advances and applications in cancer diagnosis. OncoTargets and Therapy. 2016;**9**:7355-7365. DOI: 10.2147/OTT.S99807

[10] Bacher U, Kohlmann A, Haferlach T. Perspectives of gene expression profiling for diagnosis and therapy in haematological malignancies. Briefings in Functional Genomics & Proteomics. 2009;**8**(3):184-193. DOI: 10.1093/bfgp/elp011. Epub: May 27, 2009

[11] Gallipoli P, Giotopoulos G, Huntly BJ. Epigenetic regulators as promising therapeutic targets in acute myeloid leukemia. Therapeutic Advances in Hematology. 2015;**6**(3):103-119. DOI: 10.1177/2040620715577614

[12] Burke MJ, Bhatla T. Epigenetic modifications in pediatric acute lymphoblastic leukemia. Frontiers in Pediatrics. 2014;**2**:42. DOI: 10.3389/fped.2014.00042. eCollection 2014

[13] Charmsaz S, Scott AM, Boyd AW. Targeted therapies in hematological malignancies using therapeutic monoclonal antibodies against Eph family receptors. Experimental Hematology. 2017;**54**:31-39. DOI: 10.1016/j.exphem.2017.07.003. Epub: July 24, 2017

[14] Lohr JG, Stojanov P, Carter SL, Multiple Myeloma Research Consortium, et al. Widespread genetic heterogeneity in multiple myeloma: Implications for targeted therapy. Cancer Cell. 2014;**25**:91-101. DOI: 10.1016/j.ccr.2013.12.015

[15] Harada H, Harada Y. Recent advances in myelodysplastic syndromes: Molecular pathogenesis and its implications for targeted therapies. Cancer Science. 2015;**106**:329-336. DOI: 10.1111/cas.12614. Epub: February 25, 2015

[16] Küppers R. Molecular biology of Hodgkin lymphoma. Hematology. American Society of Hematology. Education Program. 2009;**1**:491-496. DOI: 10.1182/asheducation-2009.1.491

[17] Miles RR, Shah RK, Frazer JK. Molecular genetics of childhood, adolescent and young adult non-Hodgkin lymphoma. British Journal of Haematology. 2016;**173**:582-596. DOI: 10.1111/bjh.14011

[18] Cazzola M. Introduction to a review series: The 2016 revision of the WHO classification of tumors of hematopoietic and lymphoid tissues. Blood. 2016;**127**(20):2361-2364. DOI: 10.1182/blood-2016-03-657379. Epub: April 11, 2016

[19] Passamonti F, Mora B, Maffioli M. New molecular genetics in the diagnosis and treatment of myeloproliferative neoplasms. Current Opinion in Hematology. 2016;**23**(2):137-143. DOI: 10.1097/MOH.0000000000000218

[20] Moss P. BTK inhibition saunters to the front of the line in CLL. The Hematologist. 2017;**14**:1

[21] Kasamon YL, de Claro RA, Wang Y, et al. FDA approval summary: Nivolumab for the treatment of relapsed or progressive classical Hodgkin lymphoma. The Oncologist. 2017;**22**(5):585-591. DOI: 10.1634/theoncologist.2017-0004. Epub: April 24, 2017

[22] Sorge CE, McDaniel JK, Xavier AC. Targeted therapies for the treatment of pediatric non-Hodgkin lymphomas: Present and future. Pharmaceuticals (Basel). 2016;**9**(2):pii: E28. DOI: 10.3390/ph9020028

[23] Pettirossi V, Santi A, Imperi E, et al. BRAF inhibitors reverse the unique molecular signature and phenotype of hairy cell leukemia and exert potent antileukemic activity. Blood. 2015;**125**(8):1207-1216. DOI: 10.1182/blood-2014-10-603100. Epub: December 5, 2014

[24] Benjamin H, Yiping Y. New developments in immunotherapy for lymphoma. Cancer Biology & Medicine. 2018;**15**(3):189-209. DOI: 10.20892/j.issn.2095-3941.2018.0037

[25] Olsen E, Duvic M, Frankel A, et al. Pivotal phase III trial of two dose levels of denileukin diftitox for the treatment of cutaneous T-cell lymphoma. Journal of Clinical Oncology. 2001;**19**:376-388. DOI: 10.1200/JCO.2001.19.2.376

[26] Shih LB, Lu HH, Xuan H, et al. Internalization and intracellular processing of anti-B-cell lymphoma monoclonal antibody, LL2. International Journal of Cancer. 1994;**56**:538-545

[27] DiNardo CD, Ravandi F, Agresta S, et al. Characteristics, clinical outcome, and prognostic significance of IDH mutations in AML. American Journal of Hematology. 2015;**90**(8):732-736. DOI: 10.1002/ajh.24072

[28] The ASCO Post. Enasidenib in IDH2-Mutant Relapsed or Refractory Acute Myeloid Leukemia. 2018. Retrieved from: http://ascopost.com/issues/february-10-2018/enasidenib-in-idh2-mutant-relapsed-or-refractory-acute-myeloid-leukemia/

[29] Stone RM, Fischer T, Paquette R, et al. Phase IB study of the FLT3 kinase inhibitor midostaurin with chemotherapy in younger newly diagnosed adult patients with acute myeloid leukemia. Leukemia. 2012;**26**(9):2061-2068. DOI: 10.1038/leu.2012.115

[30] Ginaldi L, De Martinis M, Matutes E, et al. Levels of expression of CD52 in normal and leukemic B and T cells: Correlation with in vivo therapeutic responses to Campath-1H. Leukemia Research. 1998;**22**:185-191

[31] Russ A, Hua AB, Montfort WR, et al. "Don't eat me" signal of CD47-SIRPα in hematological malignancies, an in-depth review. Blood Reviews. 2018;**32**:480-489

[32] Carnahan J, Stein R, Qu ZX, et al. Epratuzumab, a CD22-targeting recombinant humanized antibody with a different mode of action from rituximab. Blood Reviews. 2018;**32**(6):480-489. DOI: 10.1016/j.blre.2018.04.005. Epub: April 14, 2018

[33] Kantarjian Hagop M, DeAngelo Daniel J, Matthias S, et al. Inotuzumab ozogamicin versus standard therapy for acute lymphoblastic leukemia. The New England Journal of Medicine. 2016;**375**:740-753. DOI: 10.1056/NEJMoa1509277

[34] Dreyling M, Santoro A, Mollica L, et al. Abstract CT149: Copanlisib in patients with relapsed or refractory indolent B-cell lymphoma: Primary results of the pivotal Chronos-1 study. Cancer Research. 2017;**77**(13 Suppl):49

[35] Miklos D, Cutler CS, Arora M, et al. Ibrutinib for chronic graft-versus-host disease after failure of prior therapy. Blood. 2017;**130**(21):2243-2250. DOI: 10.1182/blood-2017-07-793786. Epub: September 18, 2017

[36] Donald Harvey R. New drug updates in hematologic malignancies: CAR-T, targeted therapeutics, and other agents. Journal of the Advanced Practitioner in Oncology. 2018;**9**(3):282-286

[37] Duong CP, Yong CS, Kershaw MH, et al. Cancer immunotherapy utilizing gene-modified T cells: From the bench to the clinic. Molecular Immunology. 2015;**67**(2 Pt A):46-57. DOI: 10.1016/j.molimm.2014.12.009. Epub: January 13, 2015

[38] Bonini C, Mondino A. Adoptive T-cell therapy for cancer: The era of engineered T cells. European Journal of Immunology. 2015;**45**(9):2457-2469. DOI: 10.1002/eji.201545552. Epub: August 21, 2015

[39] Salmikangas P, Kinsella N, Chamberlain P. Chimeric antigen receptor T-Cells (CAR T-Cells) for cancer immunotherapy—Moving target for industry? Pharmaceutical Research. 2018;**35**(8):152. DOI: 10.1007/s11095-018-2436-z

[40] Gratwohl A, Baldomero H, Horisberger B, et al. Current trends in hematopoietic stem cell transplantation in Europe. Blood. 2002;**100**:2374-2386. DOI: 10.1182/blood-2002-03-0675

Chapter 2

Advances in Acute Myeloid Leukemia Stem Cells

Xiaoxiao Yang, Xuewen Xu, Yanfang Liu, Aihua Gong, Dongqing Wang, Xiang Liao and Haitao Zhu

Abstract

As a common hematological malignant tumor, acute leukemia is believed to originate from a subpopulation of special cancer cells, named cancer stem cells. Cancer stem cells are recognized to be the main source of tumor origin, multidrug resistance, metastasis, and recurrence. Leukemic stem cells (LSCs) were first identified and confirmed to play an important role in the occurrence and development of leukemia. In this article, we summarize the following content: special markers and sorting methods for acute myeloid leukemia stem cells and the role of cancer stem cells in treatment resistance, metastasis and invasion, recurrence, and target treatment of acute leukemia.

Keywords: acute myeloid leukemia, cancer stem cells, leukemic stem cells, treatment resistance, metastasis

1. Introduction

Acute myeloid leukemia (AML) is a group of heterogeneous diseases characterized by the uncontrolled proliferation of myeloid precursor cells and the replacement of normal hematopoiesis in the bone marrow. According to the latest survey, AML is a common cancer in adults and the second most common leukemia in children, with relatively higher rates observed in countries with high Human Development Index in North America, Oceania, and Europe [1]. The annual incidence rate of AML in the world is 2.25/100,000, and the incidence increases with age. The number is below 1/100,000 for people under 30 years of age and 17/100,000 for those above 75 years of age. Therefore, AML is actually a middle-aged and elderly disease, accounting for 80–90% of adult acute leukemia, but only accounts for 15–20% of children leukemia. Men have a higher incidence of AML than women, especially in North America, Oceania, Europe, and Asia. Epidemiology shows that environmental, occupational, and genetic factors are closely related to the pathogenesis of AML. Genetic changes in tumor cloning lead to a cascade of reactivity at the molecular level that cause abnormal proliferation and differentiation of malignant cells and inhibit normal hematopoiesis.

Tumorigenesis has been long known to resemble organogenesis and is a heterogeneous process involving many phenotypically and functionally different cells. The cancer stem cell (CSC) concept was first reported more than a century ago and refers to a very small subset of relatively quiescent cells in the tumor that are endowed with the ability to self-renew and differentiate into non-stem daughter cells that make the bulk of tumor [2]. Leukemic stem cells (LSCs) were first identified and confirmed to play an important role in the occurrence and development of leukemia. In 1994, Lapidot et al. reported that AML contains LSC. It is believed that only 0.1–1% cells have the ability to produce AML [3]. The researchers transplanted sublethal doses of $CD34^{+}CD38^{+}$ and $CD34^{+}CD38^{-}$ subpopulations isolated from the bone marrow of a patient with AML into non-obese diabetic mice with severe combined immunodeficiency disease (NOD/SCID mice). After 4–8 weeks, human AML cells isolated from the engrafted murine bone marrow expression both of $CD34^{+}CD38^{-}$. The recipient mouse, re-implanted with $CD34^{+}CD38^{-}$ cells, could survive and pass to the next generation. The researchers also found $CD34^{+}CD38^{-}$ cells can induce various subtypes of leukemia other than M3, thus indicating that this subpopulation of cells has stem cell-like strong self-renewal and reproductive ability. In 1997, Bonnet et al. confirmed the presence of LSC in NOD/SCID mice [4]. Inoculation of 10^6 LSCs resulted in the formation of human AML in animals; this finding suggested that the "source of all evils" is LSC (**Figure 1**) [5]. Since then, the existence of LSC has been recognized, which is a significant milestone. The presence of LSC has been confirmed not only in hematological malignancies but also in some solid tumors.

Although LCSs were identified and thought to be the main cause of leukemia origin, recurrence, and drug resistance, there is still controversy regarding the origin of this distinct population [6]. Several hypotheses have been proposed with regard to the origin of LCS: (1) from hematopoietic stem cells (HSCs) [7]; (2) from partially differentiated hematopoietic progenitor cells [8]; (3) from blood vascular stem cells and granulocyte macrophage precursors (GMPs) [9–11]; and (4) from relatively mature leukemia cells [12]. Although the number of LSCs is small, LSCs have the same potential for self-renewal, multidirectional differentiation, and unlimited proliferation, resistance to cell death, multidrug resistance, metastasis, and recurrence. Because they can escape inhibition by most chemotherapeutic

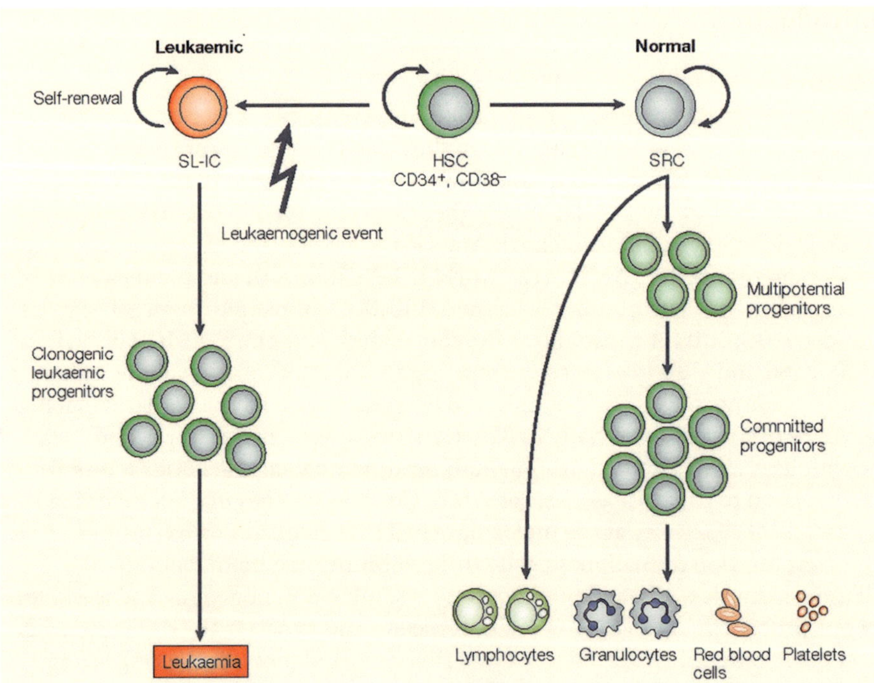

Figure 1.
Comparison of the normal and AML human hematopoietic systems.

drugs, LSCs in a relatively quiescent state can be latent for a long time. Once the conditions are appropriate, such as a certain stimulus into the cell cycle, they can escape the immune surveillance of the body, thus showing unlimited proliferation. Therefore, relevant research and analysis on the biological characteristics of LSCs may provide new ideas for therapeutic regimens. The discovery of LSCs has broadened the treatment of leukemia, and targeted therapy of related signaling pathways and niche may become a new research hotspot.

2. Expression of special surface markers in LSCs

Bonnet et al. revealed that the $CD34^{+}CD38^{-}$ subpopulation is similar to normal HSCs with surface markers and can be used to identify cells with unlimited proliferation and differentiation in AML [4]. Subsequent studies have shown that the surface markers of LSCs are extremely complex and vary from person to person. Previous experiments have demonstrated that in some cases, subpopulations of cells with different phenotypes have LSC activity [13–15]. CD34 and CD38 are no longer specific markers that define LSCs. Recent studies have identified various new markers such as CLL-1, CD96, TIM3, CD47, CD32, and CD25. The current study summarizes some of the specific markers expressed by LSCs (**Table 1**) [16] and has been utilized to successfully validate LSCs in recent clinical trials [17].

2.1 CLL-1

C-type lectin domain family 12 member A (CLL1, also known as CLEC12A) positive cells show high tumorigenicity in immunodeficient mice, indicating that this cell subpopulation has the characteristics of LSCs. Moreover, the side population cells enriched in LSCs isolated by flow cytometry from patients with AML also express CLL-1 [18]. Jiang et al. have reported that CLL1-antibody-drug conjugate (CLL1-ADC) could become an attractive target therapy for AML [19]. The use of a

Marker	Expression on LSC	Reference
CD34	+/	[4, 13]
CD38	+/−	[4, 12, 13]
CD90	−/+	[16]
CD123	++	[16, 22]
CD45RA	+	[15]
CD33	++	[90, 91]
CD13	++	[15]
CD44	++	[15]
CLL-1	+	[17, 18]
CD96	++	[16, 19]
TIM3	++	[15]
CD47	++	[23–26]
CD32	+	[27–30]
CD25	+	[27–31]

Table 1.
Summary of cell surface marker expression on AML LSCs.

DNA-binding payload in CLL1-ADC is critical because such a payload affords the ADC the ability to kill both proliferative and quiescent cells, thus making CLL1-ADC a very compelling candidate for the treatment of patients with AML.

2.2 CD96

CD96 is a member of the immunoglobulin superfamily, a transmembrane glycoprotein, and a T-cell surface-specific receptor 6. By using blood samples from 55 patients with AML, Du et al. found that CD96 (>10%)-enriched patients showed a poor response to chemotherapy [20]. Of note, CD96 was proved to be an efficient identical marker of LSCs in $CD34^{+}CD38^{-}$ groups.

2.3 CD44

CD44 is a surface glycoprotein and a receptor for hyaluronic acid, which is mainly involved in cell-cell interaction, adhesion, and migration [16]. $CD44^{+}$ cancer cells show higher sphere-forming ability and treatment resistance. CD44 is not only a special marker of LSC, but it is also a key regulator of LSC function that is essential for homing of LSCs to microenvironmental niches and for maintaining LSCs in a primitive state.

2.4 CD123 (IL3Rα)

Approximately 45% of AML cells that overexpress CD123 have higher proliferative activity and are more tolerant to apoptotic stimulation. Clinical studies have also demonstrated patients overexpressing CD123 usually have a poor prognosis. Williams et al. found that NK-92 preferentially inhibits leukemic stem cells compared with bulk leukemia cells [21]. NK-92 combined with the anti-CD123 antibody, 7G3, enhanced survival in a primary AML xenograft model when compared with control arms. Some other IL3R antibodies (DT388IL3, CSL362, and MGD006) can significantly prolong the survival rate of patients with AML [22, 23].

2.5 CD47

CD47 is a transmembrane glycoprotein that is widely expressed in human tissues. CD47 also functions as a marker of "self" on host cells within an organism. When expressed, CD47 binds to SIRPα on the surface of circulating immune cells to deliver an inhibitory "don't eat me" signal [24]. Higher expression of CD47 has been demonstrated in LSCs [25, 26]. Anti-CD47 antibody treatment has also been shown to act synergistically with cytarabine (Ara-C) chemotherapy in a model of AML. While Ara-C effectively eliminated TSP-1 cancer cells in the proliferative phase, anti-CD47 antibodies were putatively able to target quiescent LSCs that were not susceptible to Ara-C treatment but highly expressed CD47 [27].

2.6 CD25 and CD32

Saito et al. conducted microarray analysis and found that CD25 and CD35 were expressed on quiescent LSCs, but not on HSCs [28]. The activation of CD25, namely IL2Rα, can control cell proliferation, survival, and differentiation. CD32 is a member of the Fc-gamma receptor family and is mainly found on immune cells. Transplantation of $CD34^{+}CD38^{-}CD25^{+}$ cells and $CD34^{+}CD38^{-}CD32^{+}$ cells into NO/SCID mice can trigger leukemia and resistance to cytarabine. It has been reported that overexpression of CD25 in AML cells may be caused by the activation of STAT5 and MYC [29, 30]. Gönen et al. analyzed the correlation between the expression of CD25 (IL-2 receptor alpha) and prognosis in 657 patients with primary AML (≤60 years old); they concluded that CD25 can be used as a biomarker for poor prognosis of AML [31]. Cerny et al. also indicated that CD25 expression can be used as an indicator to predict early treatment failure in AML [32].

3. LSCs are the source of treatment resistance

The most fundamental reason for the relapse of AML is the existence of LSCs. It is necessary to investigate the key mechanisms of resistance of LSCs to the current treatment strategy for effective clearance of LSC.

3.1 LSCs are mostly in the G0 quiescent phase

Dean et al. showed that 96% of LSCs are in the G0 phase of the cell cycle [33]. Chemotherapeutic drugs acting on the cell cycle or on rapidly differentiating cells can inhibit only differentiated mature leukemia cells, while LSCs in the G0 phase cannot be completely inhibited because they do not divide. Once they are properly stimulated to re-enter the cell cycle, they will continue to proliferate and differentiate into daughter leukemia cells, thus causing recurrence. According to some studies, LSCs are much less sensitive to daunorubicin and cytarabine than differentiated leukemia cells.

3.2 LSCs highly express multidrug resistance genes and proteins

The expression of multidrug resistance genes on the surface of LSCs can induce the production of various membrane transporters that can pump a variety of chemotherapeutic drugs out of the cell, which results in lowering the concentration of the drug in the cancer cells. The ABC membrane transporter plays a pivotal role in this drug efflux process. The ABC transporter, namely the ATP-binding cassette transporter, has an ATP-dependent drug-release function [34]. The most representative multidrug resistance genes are ABCB1, ABCC1, and ABCG2, which encode P-glycoproteins (P-gp, P-170, and MDR1), multidrug resistance protein (MRP), and breast cancer resistance protein (BCRP), respectively. BCRP is preferentially expressed in $CD34^{+}CD38^{-}$ LSCs. The intracellular drug concentration after BCRP inhibition is increased, but it is much lower than that of cells expressing only BCRP. Therefore, it is indicated that the drug resistance of LSC is related to the interaction of multiple drug resistance proteins. Some other reports have revealed that LSC has higher MDR1, MRP, BCRP, and lung resistance related protein (LRP) expression relative to HSC, thus giving LSC a stronger drug resistance advantage. The high expression of multidrug resistance gene in LSCs is the main mechanism by which LSCs exhibit primary resistance to chemotherapeutic drugs [35, 36].

3.3 LSC display higher self-renewal ability

Hope et al. proved that LSCs have self-renewal ability, which is one of the most prominent features of CSCs [37]. The self-renewal ability of LSCs may be one of the key factors that promote the development and metastasis of leukemia, and the molecular regulation mechanism is very complicated. Bmi-1 is a member of the PcG (polycomb group) transcriptional repressor family and is an essential factor in maintaining HSC self-renewal. Raffel et al. showed that miR-126 overexpression renders AML cells more resistant to standard chemotherapy and that treatment of primary AML cells results in the enrichment of LSC-like cells with increased miR-126 levels [38]. Moreover, leukemic cells with high miR-126 expression were selected in refractory patients after induction chemotherapy, thus correlating high miR-126 levels to LSCs and therapy resistance. miR-126 knockdown leads to the expansion of HSCs but impaired maintenance of LSCs, and its overexpression promotes LSC self-renewal, which is inhibited in HSCs [39, 40]. In addition, all genes and signaling pathways that contribute to HSC self-renewal may be involved in LSCs, such as Wnt, Notch, HOX, and Shh. Recent studies have revealed that the activation of the Shh signaling pathway in LSCs by upregulation of SMO is essential for LSC survival maintenance [41, 42].

3.4 The special microenvironment (niche)

The receptors CXCR4 on the LSC membrane and CXCL12 in the bone marrow microenvironment are required for LSC to maintain dormancy, self-renewal, differentiation, growth, and homing. However, targeted therapy for the niche will enhance the expression of the drug pump MDR1, which induced LSC insensitive to therapy and failed to achieve the goal of reversing its resistance [43].

3.5 Multiple signaling pathway abnormalities

Recent studies have demonstrated that abnormal activation of multiple signaling pathways is one of the key mechanisms of LSC multidrug resistance, such as Sonic Hedgehog, Bmi-1, Nocth, and WNT. Among these pathways, the abnormality of Hedgehog (Hh) pathway is closely related to CSC resistance, such as increased endogenous synthesis of ligand protein Hh, loss of PCTH activity, inhibition of smoothened (SMO) signaling protein, mutation of SUFU, and overexpression of the transcription factor GLI1, thus regulating the downstream target gene and participating in the maintenance of stem cell proliferation, which are related to multiple hallmarks of tumor cell resistance [44, 45]. Studies have revealed that Hh signaling is abnormally activated in LSCs, GLI1 can induce endogenous BCL-2 expression, and the Hh pathway also up-regulates BCL-2 by activating PI3K/AKT, thus leading to apoptotic disorder and drug resistance of LSCs.

4. The role of LSCs in tumor metastasis and invasion

CSCs are thought to be the seed of tumor metastasis. CSCs that particularly express C-X-C chemokine receptor type 4 (CXCR4) preferentially disseminate [46]. The specific ligand for the CXCR4 chemokine receptor is termed matrix-derived factor-1 (SDF-1, also known as CXCL12). Both CXCR4 and SDF-1 are expressed in various tissues and cell types and regulate cell migration [47]. The SDF-1/CXCR4 axis is also involved in the migration of CSCs [48]. SDF-1 is a homeostatic chemokine secreted by stromal cells and is released into the interstitial space [49]. On the one hand, SDF-1 exerts effects through its unique physiologic cognate receptor CXCR4, which is known to mediate chemotaxis, hematopoiesis, angiogenesis, and tumor spread and metastasis. On the other hand, it also acts in a paracrine fashion on cells in the local microenvironment to stimulate directional migration of hematopoietic and nonhematopoietic normal and malignant cells [50–52]. Li et al. found that HERG K^+ channels were widely expressed in primary leukemic cells but not in normal lymphocytes [53, 54]. Blocking HERG K^+ channels by applying its specific inhibitor in hematopoietic cell lines and primary leukemic cells significantly reduced the migration of leukemic cells induced by SDF-1; this indicated a role for HERG K^+ channels in the progression of leukemia.

Currently, there is a lack of direct evidence linking LSCs to metastasis. There are some sporadic reports that LSCs may play a role in metastasis. In patients with AML, low levels of CXCR4 expression have been shown to be associated with better prognosis, longer recurrence-free period, and overall survival. It has also been suggested that CXCR4 is an independent prognostic predictor of disease recurrence and survival [55]. Another study has shown that overexpression of C-myc, Bmi-1, Oct4, and Nanog in precancerous and cancerous cells may initiate oncogenic epithelial-mesenchymal transition and tumorigenesis, which plays important roles in the genesis of CSCs, malignant tumor initiation and progression, cancer metastasis, and drug resistance [56]. Compared with the parental cells, chemotherapy-resistant $MOLT4^+$ cells expressed much higher levels of the stem cell surface marker CXCR4. It was found that the expression of CXCR4, related to tumor cell homing and migration, was significantly higher in $MOLT4^+$ cells than in $MOLT4^-$ cells. In addition, hMDSCs-MOLT4 cells seem to have a strong invasive potential in vivo, as demonstrated by strong interstitial and vascular tissues in tumor tissue sections.

It was confirmed that the niche was involved in metastasis. With respect to HSCs, two distinct niches have been defined: the osteoblastic niche and the vascular niche [57–59]. Tabe et al. hypothesized the presence of a "metastatic niche" that facilitates the survival, proliferation, and metastasis of LSCs [60]. Yang et al. demonstrated that vascular endothelial growth factor receptor 1 (VEGFR1) was involved in the initiation of a premetastatic niche and that cells expressing VEGFR1 home to tumor-specific premetastatic sites and form cellular clusters before the arrival of tumor cell clusters [61]. They can alter the local microenvironment and lead to the activation of integrins and chemokines. After treatment with anti-VEGFR1 antibodies, the supportive premetastatic cell clusters were abolished and metastasis was prevented, which indicated the importance of a metastatic niche.

5. The role of LSCs in tumor proliferation and anti-apoptosis

Various signaling pathways that stimulate proliferation or inhibit apoptosis are known to aberrant activate LSCs.

5.1 Hedgehog pathway

The Hh pathway is a highly conserved pathway that regulates the proliferation, migration, and differentiation of cells during development [62, 63]. Three distinct ligands, namely Sonic (Shh), Indian (Ihh), and Desert (Dhh) Hedgehog, exist in humans. Upon ligand binding to the receptor pat (Ptch), inhibition of smoothened (Smo) receptor is relieved. Smo then activates members of the Gli family of zinc-finger transcription factors, translocating them to the nucleus to regulate the transcription of Hh target genes including Gli1, Gli2, and Ptch, and regulators of cell proliferation and survival [64–66].

The Hh pathway promotes cell proliferation mainly by regulating cell cycle. Its regulation mechanism is as follows [67]: (1) Cyclin D1 and cyclin D2 act as downstream target genes for the transcription factor GLI1 and are involved in cell cycle G1 to S phase transformation; (2) PTCH regulates the activity of cyclin B, which is part of the mitosis promoting factor (MPF) compound. MPF is required for cell entry from the G2 phase to the M phase; and (3) SMO proteins block cellular dormancy by modulating P21, a cyclin-dependent inhibitory protein.

The Hh signaling pathway regulates apoptosis mainly through the following mechanisms: (1) Regulate the activity of the BCL-2 family. The BCL-2 family is divided into anti-apoptotic proteins (such as BCL-2, BCL-XL, and MCL-1) and pro-apoptotic proteins (such as BAX, BAD, and BAK). The ratio between the two types of proteins will directly affect the stability of the mitochondrial membrane and is the most important regulator of the mitochondrial apoptosis pathway. Overexpression of BCL-2, an increase in the ratio of BCL-2 to BAD, leading to defects in mitochondrial apoptosis, is one of the important mechanisms for LSC multidrug resistance and poor prognosis of AML [68]. BCL-2 is the target gene downstream of the Hh pathway, and Hh pathway blockers can induce apoptosis by downregulating BCL-2 [69]. Kobune et al. found that cyclopamine induces apoptosis of drug-resistant $CD34^+$ AML cells by downregulating BCL-2 and makes them sensitive to Ara-C [70]. MCL1 has also emerged as a mechanism of resistance to apoptosis and to BCL-2/BCL-XL inhibitors, and therefore, it is considered as a potential therapeutic target [71]. (2) Regulation of tumor necrosis factor-related apoptosis-inducing ligand (TRAIL) mediated apoptosis. TRAIL-R3 is a blank receptor that lacks a functional death region and is highly expressed in $CD34^+CD38^-$ LSCs; the downregulation of TRAIL-R3 increases apoptosis [72]. (3) Regulation of FAS protein express in the death receptor pathway. Studies have found that the Hh pathway inhibitor GDC-0449 promotes tumor stem cell apoptosis by upregulating FAS protein [73].

5.2 NF-κB pathway

NF-κB is a significant transcriptional activator located upstream of the IRF-1 gene. It is aberrantly activated by LSCs. NF-κB not only inhibits apoptosis but also regulating the expression of cytokine genes. Furthermore, apoptosis can be inhibited by inducing and upregulating antiapoptotic genes. Therefore, NF-κB plays an essential role in maintaining LSC growth and survival. Inhibition of this signaling pathway not only promotes LSC apoptosis but also enhances the sensitivity of LSCs to chemotherapeutic drugs [74, 75]. At present, the targeted drugs for NF-κB are mainly proteasome inhibitors MG-132 and Bortezomib (VELCADE, PS-341), which can better target LSCs without any significant effect on normal HSC. It was reported that PTL can specifically induce apoptosis of LSCs by inhibiting NF-κB activity. At present, the PTL analog DMAP has been developed, and its experimental effect is remarkable [76, 77].

5.3 PI3K/Akt pathway

The PI3K/Akt pathway is an intracellular pathway that plays a critical role in apoptosis and cancer, whose components are often altered in cancer, leading to dysregulated apoptosis and chemoresistance [78]. Chen et al. demonstrated that the PI3K inhibitor LY294002 can directly target LSCs without adverse reactions to normal HSCs, and they found that PI3K and NF-κB may coexist in the same signaling pathway [79]. Further, it has been reported that the mammalian target of rapamycin (mTOR) is a substrate for PI3K that regulates the survival of LCSs after etoposide treatment. Mise et al. showed that the inhibitory effect of rapamycin on mTOR significantly reduced the survival rate of AML cells, and rapamycin enhanced the effect of etoposide on these cells [80]. It is found that PTEN that negatively regulates the PI3K pathway and is essential for maintaining normal hematopoiesis [81]. However, PTEN deletion has no significant effect on HSC differentiation survival, while PTEN deletion in LSCs can lead to the production and proliferation of LSCs. In addition, rapamycin, an inhibitor of the PI3K pathway downstream regulator of mTOR was found to inhibit LSCs and protect against normal HSC failure.

6. Treatment avenue for LSC

6.1 Niche of LSCs

Niche is involved in stem cell self-renewal, survival, chemotherapy tolerance, and metastasis of leukemia cells [82]. In the mice model, it was found that the homing of HSCs to the bone marrow is regulated by chemokine CXCL12 expressed in mesenchymal stem cells, and its receptor is CXCR4 [83]. Inhibition of CXCL12-CXCR4 interaction helps to reduce chemotaxis, thus affecting the movement, adhesion, and metastasis of LSCs. In vitro studies have shown that the anti-leukemia active peptide CXCR4 inhibitor LY2510924, as a single agent or in combination chemotherapy, can rapidly and permanently destroy the CXCL12-CXCR4 axis, thereby inhibiting the proliferation of AML cells and leading to apoptosis [84]. Fully human IgG4 monoclonal antibody BMS-936564 against CXCR4 showed high safety and antitumor activity in relapsed and refractory patients with AML [85]. However, because of the similar biological properties of LSCs and HSCs, the non-selection of related inhibitors has become another major clinical problem.

In addition to participating in the hematopoietic function, the bone marrow niche is also an important place for the presence of immune cells. There is a group of activated leukemia-specific immune cells in leukemia bone marrow, and regulatory T cell (Treg) is one of the important members [86]. Fujisaki et al. found that hematopoietic stem/progenitor cells and Treg can coexist on the endosteum of murine bone marrow, and HSPC disappears shortly after Treg cell depletion [87]. This experiment successfully demonstrated the involvement of Treg cells in the formation of bone marrow niche. Treg is a dynamic cell population that regulates the immune response. Stem cells evade immune surveillance by recruiting Treg cells and using their regulatory functions [88]. Therefore, it is speculated that these cells will likely become new targets for eliminating LSCs (**Figure 2**) [89].

6.2 LSCs-related signaling pathways

Leukemia is characterized by selective overgrowth of LSCs and interferes with the differentiation of HSCs. Chemotherapy kills rapidly dividing cancer cells, but does not eliminate reservoirs of LSCs that cause relapse. LSCs have a variety of regulatory abnormal signaling pathways, including WNT/β-catenin, JAK/STAT, PI3K/AKT, RAS, NF-κB, and Notch. WNT is involved in the maintenance of properties of LSCs. Riether et al. discovered that tyrosine kinase inhibitors induced CD70 expression on LSCs during targeted drug therapy, while CD70 inhibited WNT/β-catenin signaling pathway [90]. STAT is an important transcription factor regulating cell growth, proliferation, and inhibition of apoptosis. Activation of the JAK/STAT signaling pathway is associated with sustained activation of the proto-oncogene AHI-1 in CD34 cells, regulating CML-LSC autonomous growth in vitro and inducing leukemia [91].

In recent years, studies on micro-RNA and transcription factors in leukemia patients have become increasingly mature. For example, the transcription factor MYC can inhibit the expression of the shared target gene FLT3 by miR-15a-5p, and FLT3 plays a crucial role in activating the STAT5A pathway and promoting tumor cell proliferation [92, 93], but its specific mechanism of influence on the development of tumor remains to be further investigated. Targeted drugs in mounting numbers for LSCs signaling pathways are being developed, but most of them are still in the stage of animal experiments, and more research is needed to determine the safety and efficacy in humans.

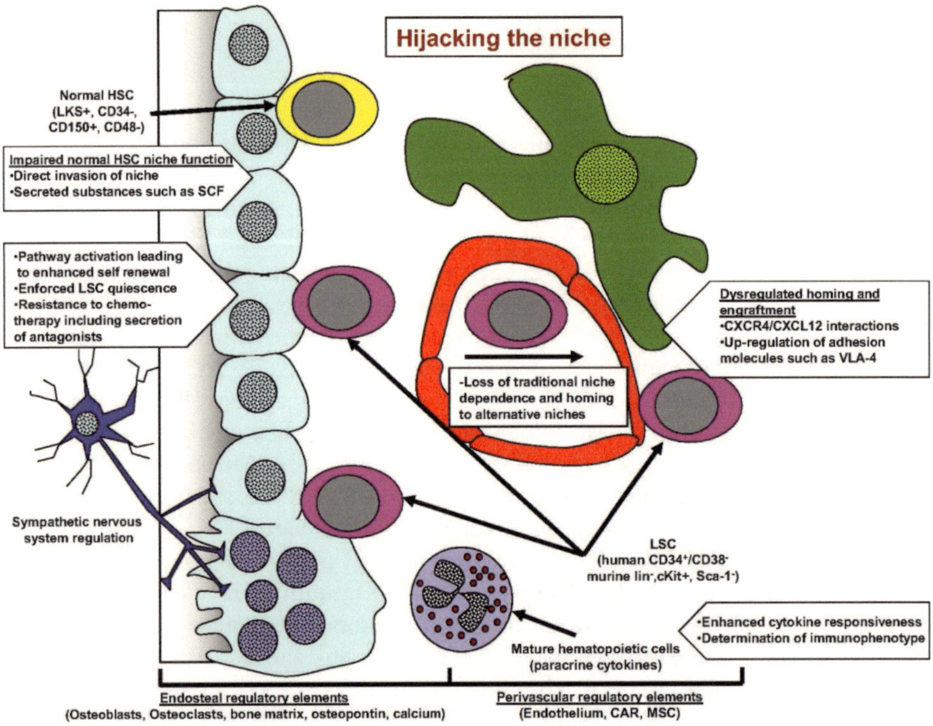

Figure 2.
The niche of leukemic stem cell. The niche provides support for self-renewal, quiescence, homing, engraftment, and proliferative potential for HSCs. LSCs may impair the function of the normal HSC niche. In addition, LSCs can infiltrate these niches and may hijack these normal homeostatic processes.

6.3 Cell cycle of LSCs

In patients with drug resistance, most of their LSCs are in the quiescent phase (G0 phase) and therefore cannot be effectively eliminated by chemotherapy. Hence, some people consider that LSCs in stationary phase can be eliminated by two-step method: (1) Stimulate LSCs from the G0 phase into the cell cycle proliferation and then use specific tumor-targeted therapeutic drugs to eliminate LSCs and (2) Let LSCs stay in the G0 phase. It is worth noting that although the cells in the G0 phase are dormant, they have the ability to proliferate; thus, this can only delay survival and avoid recurrence. Experiments in vitro have shown that cyclin-dependent kinase (CDK6) can be involved in the regulation of cell cycle, and inhibition of CDK6 may cause leukemia stem cells to dormant and inhibit cell proliferation [94].

6.4 Immunophenotype of LSCs

Several immunophenotypes of LSCs have been identified, such as CD34, CD38, CD123, CD117, CD71, CD44, HLA-DR, TIM3, CLL-1, CD96, CD47, CD32 and CD25. Although these surface molecules are not expressed in all LSCs, their high expression may lead to a significant deterioration of the disease prognosis. It is also because of the difference in markers and functions between LSCs and HSCs that targeted therapy for leukemia stem cells is possible. CD33 is the first AML targeted therapeutic antigen approved by the US FDA, which is highly expressed in AML but not in normal HSCs. The monoclonal anti-tumor drug Gemtuzumab ozogamicin, consisting of the CD33 antibody, hP67.6, and the cytotoxic drug, is a good candidate for selective killing of $CD33^+$ LSCs [95]. In addition, in recent years, tumor-specific chimeric antigen receptor T-cell immunotherapy (CART) against $CD33^+$ cells has become increasingly popular [96]. Busfield et al. detected that the anti-CD123 monoclonal antibody CSL362 has a good tumor cell killing effect in the AML mouse model [22].

Although the current monoclonal antibodies against the LSCs phenotype have achieved initial clinical success, it is undeniable that LSCs are diverse among different patients, and even in the same individual, the phenotypic differences are quite different. This brings new challenges to clinical treatment. Moreover, studies have shown that in patients with newly diagnosed AML, the distribution of LSCs is uniform and the number is small, but once the patient relapses after chemotherapy, the number of LSCs can be significantly increased, and some new phenotypes appear [97]. The phenotypic changes in LSCs at different stages of the same patient's disease also lead to difficulties in clinical application of this targeted LSC immunophenotypic treatment strategy. Therefore, the current targeted therapy based on this strategy is still in the exploration stage, and the development of related drugs is significantly limited due to the plasticity of the immunophenotype of LSCs.

7. Summary

LSCs play an important role in the origin, recurrence, and drug resistance of leukemia. Although the current research on LSCs has made some progress, the biological characteristics of LSCs and its mechanism in the pathogenesis of leukemia remain unclear, and the treatment strategy for targeted clearance of LSCs is still in its infancy. Therefore, clarifying its biological characteristics and developing drugs for targeted therapy of LSCs is an important direction for leukemia research in future.

Acknowledgements

The authors acknowledge financial support from the National Natural Science Foundation of China (Grant no. 81502663), Social Development Foundation of Zhenjiang City (Grant no. SH2018063), Six talent peals project of Jiangsu Province (Grant no.WSW-039), Six for one project of Jiangsu Province (Grant no. LGY2018093), Young medical talents of Jiangsu (Grant no. QNRC2016833).

Author details

Xiaoxiao Yang[1], Xuewen Xu[1], Yanfang Liu[2], Aihua Gong[3], Dongqing Wang[1], Xiang Liao[4] and Haitao Zhu[1*]

1 Central Laboratory of Radiology, Affiliated Hospital of Jiangsu University, Zhenjiang, China

2 Department of Central Laboratory, The First People's Hospital of Zhenjiang, Zhenjiang, China

3 School of Medicine, Jiangsu University, Zhenjiang, China

4 Jinling Hospital, Nanjing University, Nanjing, China

*Address all correspondence to: zhht25@163.com

References

[1] Miranda-Filho A, Piñeros M, Ferlay J, et al. Epidemiological patterns of leukaemia in 184 countries: A population-based study. Lancet Hematology. 2018;**5**(1):e14-e24. DOI: 10.1016/S2352-3026(17)30232-6

[2] Kizaki M. Molecular pathogenesis of leukemia and leukemic stem cells (LSCs). International Journal of Hematology. 2018;**109**(1):3-4. DOI: 10.1007/s12185-018-2550-z

[3] Lapidot T, Sirard C, Vormoor J, et al. A cell initiating human acute myeloid leukaemia after transplantation into SCID mice. Nature. 1994;**367**(6464): 645-648. DOI: 10.1038/367645a0

[4] Bonnet D, Dick JE. Human acute myeloid leukemia is organized as a hierarchy that originates from a primitive hematopoietic cell. Nature Medicine. 1997;**3**(7):730-737. DOI: 10.1038/nm0797-730

[5] Huntly BJ, Gilliland DG. Leukaemia stem cells and the evolution of cancer-stem-cell research. Nature Reviews Cancer. 2005;**5**(4):311-321. DOI: 10.1038/nrc1592

[6] Shlush LI, Mitchell A, Heisler L, et al. Tracing the origins of relapse in acute myeloid leukaemia to stem cells. Nature. 2017;**547**(7661):104-108. DOI: 10.1038/nature22993

[7] Le PM, Andreeff M, Battula VL. Osteogenic niche in the regulation of normal hematopoiesis and leukemogenesis. Haematologica. 2018;**103**(12):1945-1955. DOI: 10.3324/haematol.2018.197004

[8] Sugimura R, Jha DK, Han A, et al. Haematopoietic stem and progenitor cells from human pluripotent stem cells. Nature. 2017;**545**(7655):432-438. DOI: 10.1038/nature22370

[9] Duarte D, Hawkins ED, Akinduro O, et al. Inhibition of endosteal vascular niche remodeling rescues hematopoietic stem cell loss in AML. Cell Stem Cell. 2018;**22**(1):64-77.e6. DOI: 10.1016/j.stem.2017.11.006

[10] Butler JM, Rafii S. Generation of a vascular niche for studying stem cell homeostasis. Methods in Molecular Biology. 2012;**904**:221-233. DOI: 10.1007/978-1-61779-943-3_18

[11] Jamieson CHM, Ailles LE, Dylla SJ, et al. Granulocyte-macrophage progenitors as candidate leukemic stem cells in blast-crisis CML. The New England Journal of Medicine. 2004;**351**(7):657-667. DOI: 10.1056/NEJMoa040258

[12] Kazue TT, Toshiya I, Yoshihiro I, et al. Demethylating agent, 5-azacytidine, reverses differentiation of embryonic stem cells. Biochemical and Biophysical Research Communications. 2004;**323**(1):86-90. DOI: 10.1016/j.bbrc.2004.08.052

[13] Jean-Emmanuel S, Kathleen M, Robin P, et al. Human acute myelogenous leukemia stem cells are rare and heterogeneous when assayed in NOD/SCID/IL2Rγc-deficient mice. The Journal of Clinical Investigation. 2011;**121**(1):384-395. DOI: 10.1172/JCI41495

[14] Taussig DC, Vargaftig J, Miraki-Moud F, et al. Leukemia-initiating cells from some acute myeloid leukemia patients with mutated nucleophosmin reside in the CD34(−) fraction. Blood. 2010;**115**(10):1976-1984. DOI: 10.1182/blood-2009-02-206565

[15] Terwijn M, Kelder A, Snel AN, et al. Minimal residual disease detection defined as the malignant fraction of the total primitive stem cell compartment offers additional prognostic information in acute myeloid leukaemia. International Journal of Laboratory

Hematology. 2012;**34**(4):432-441. DOI: 10.1111/j.1751-553X.2012.01416.x

[16] Horton SJ, Huntly BJP. Recent advances in acute myeloid leukemia stem cell biology. Haematologica. 2012;**97**(7):966-974. DOI: 10.3324/haematol.2011.054734

[17] Antonieta CG, Elisa DA, Dafne ML, et al. Expression of CD90, CD96, CD117, and CD123 on different hematopoietic cell populations from pediatric patients with acute myeloid leukemia. Archives of Medical Research. 2014;**45**(4):343-350. DOI: 10.1016/j.arcmed.2014.04.001

[18] Tashiro H, Sauer T, Shum T, et al. Treatment of acute myeloid leukemia with T cells expressing chimeric antigen receptors directed to C-type lectin-like molecule 1. Molecular Therapy. 2017;**25**(9):2202-2213. DOI: 10.1016/j.ymthe.2017.05.024

[19] Jiang YP, Liu BY, Zheng Q, et al. CLT030, a leukemic stem cell–targeting CLL1 antibody-drug conjugate for treatment of acute myeloid leukemia. Blood Advances. 2018;**2**(14):1738-1749. DOI: 10.1182/bloodadvances.2018020107

[20] Du W, Hu Y, Lu C, et al. Cluster of differentiation 96 as a leukemia stem cell-specific marker and a factor for prognosis evaluation in leukemia. Molecular and Clinical Oncology. 2015;**3**(4):833-838. DOI: 10.3892/mco.2015.552

[21] Williams BA, Wang XH, Leyton JV, et al. $CD16^{+}$NK-92 and anti-CD123 monoclonal antibody prolongs survival in primary human acute myeloid leukemia xenografted mice. Haematologica. 2018;**103**(10):1720-1729. DOI: 10.3324/haematol.2017.187385

[22] Busfield SJ, Biondo M, Wong M, et al. Targeting of acute myeloid leukemia in vitro and in vivo with an anti-CD123 mAb engineered for optimal ADCC. Leukemia. 2014;**28**(11):2213-2221. DOI: 10.1038/leu.2014.128

[23] Chichili GR, Ling H, Hua L, et al. A CD3xCD123 bispecific DART for redirecting host T cells to myelogenous leukemia: Preclinical activity and safety in nonhuman primates. Science Translational Medicine. 2015;**7**(289):289ra82. DOI: 10.1126/scitranslmed.aaa5693

[24] Russ A, Hua AB, Montfort WR, et al. Blocking "don't eat me" signal of CD47-SIRPÎ± in hematological malignancies, an in-depth review. Blood Reviews. 2018;**32**(6):480-489. DOI: 10.1016/j.blre.2018.04.005

[25] Siddhartha J, Jamieson CHM, Pang WW, et al. CD47 is upregulated on circulating hematopoietic stem cells and leukemia cells to avoid phagocytosis. Cell. 2009;**138**(2):271-285. DOI: 10.1016/j.cell.2009.05.046

[26] Majeti R, Chao MP, Alizadeh AA, et al. CD47 is an adverse prognostic factor and therapeutic antibody target on human acute myeloid leukemia stem cells. Cell. 2009;**138**(2):286-299. DOI: 10.1016/j.cell.2009.05.045

[27] Wang Y, Yin C, Feng L, et al. Ara-C and anti-CD47 antibody combination therapy eliminates acute monocytic leukemia THP-1 cells in vivo and in vitro. Genetics and Molecular Research. 2015;**14**(2):5630-5641. DOI: 10.4238/2015.May.25.15

[28] Saito Y, Kitamura H, Hijikata A, et al. Identification of therapeutic targets for quiescent, chemotherapy-resistant human leukemia stem cells. Science Translational Medicine. 2010;**2**(17):17ra9. DOI: 10.1126/scitranslmed.3000349

[29] Schepers H, van Gosliga D, Wierenga AT, et al. STAT5 is required for long-term maintenance of normal

and leukemic human stem/progenitor cells. Blood. 2007;**110**(8):2880-2888. DOI: 10.1182/blood-2006-08-039073

[30] King B, Trimarchi T, Reavie L, et al. The ubiquitin ligase FBXW7 modulates leukemia-initiating cell activity by regulating MYC stability. Cell. 2013;**153**(7):1552-1566. DOI: 10.1016/j.cell.2013.05.041

[31] Gonen M, Sun Z, Figueroa ME, et al. CD25 expression status improves prognostic risk classification in AML independent of established biomarkers: ECOG phase 3 trial, E1900. Blood. 2012;**11**:2297-2306. DOI: 10.1182/blood-2012-02-414425

[32] Cerny J, Yu H, Ramanathan M, et al. Expression of CD25 independently predicts early treatment failure of acute myeloid leukaemia (AML). British Journal of Haematology. 2013;**160**(2):262-266. DOI: 10.1111/bjh.12109

[33] Dean M, Fojo T, Bates S. Tumor stem cells and drug resistance. Nature Reviews. Cancer. 2005;**5**:275-284. DOI: 10.1038/nrc1590

[34] Fukuda Y, Lian S, Schuetz JD. Leukemia and ABC transporters. Advances in Cancer Research. 2015;**125**:171-196. DOI: 10.1016/bs.acr.2014.10.006

[35] de Figueiredo-Pontes LL, Pintão MC, Oliveira LC, et al. Determination of P-glycoprotein, MDR-related protein 1, breast cancer resistance protein, and lung-resistance protein expression in leukemic stem cells of acute myeloid leukemia. Cytometry. Part B, Clinical Cytometry. 2010;**74**(3):163-168. DOI: 10.1002/cyto.b.20403

[36] Ho MM, Hogge DE, Ling V. MDR1 and BCRP1 expression in leukemic progenitors correlates with chemotherapy response in acute myeloid leukemia. Experimental Hematology. 2008;**36**(4):433-442. DOI: 10.1016/j.exphem.2007.11.014

[37] Hope KJ, Jin L, Dick JE. Acute myeloid leukemia originates from a hierarchy of leukemic stem cell classes that differ in self-renewal capacity. Nature Immunology. 2004;**5**(7):738-743. DOI: 10.1038/ni1080

[38] Raffel S, Trumpp A. miR-126 drives quiescence and self-renewal in leukemic stem cells. Cancer Cell. 2016;**29**(2):133-135. DOI: 10.1016/j.ccell.2016.01.007

[39] Lechman E, Gentner B, Vangalen P, et al. Attenuation of miR-126 activity expands HSC invivo without exhaustion. Cell Stem Cell. 2012;**11**(6):799-811. DOI: 10.1016/j.stem.2012.09.001

[40] Lechman E, Gentner B, Ng SK, et al. miR-126 regulates distinct self-renewal outcomes in normal and malignant hematopoietic stem cells. Cancer Cell. 2016;**29**(2):214-228. DOI: 10.1016/j.ccell.2015.12.011

[41] Deng CH, Zhang QP. Leukemia stem cells in drug resistance and metastasis. Chinese Medical Journal. 2010;**123**(7):954-960. DOI: 10.3760/cma.j.issn.0366-6999.2010.07.034

[42] Kakiuchi S, Minami Y, Miyata Y, et al. NANOG expression as a responsive biomarker during treatment with hedgehog signal inhibitor in acute myeloid leukemia. International Journal of Molecular Sciences. 2017;**18**(3):pii: E486. DOI: 10.3390/ijms18030486

[43] Paprocka M, Bielawska-Pohl A, Rossowska J, et al. MRP1 protein expression in leukemic stem cells as a negative prognostic marker in acute myeloid leukemia patients. European Journal of Haematology. 2017;**99**(5):415-422. DOI: 10.1111/ejh.12938

[44] Hay JF, Lappin K, Liberante F, et al. Integrated analysis of the

molecular action of vorinostat identifies epi-sensitised targets for combination therapy. Oncotarget. 2017;**8**(40):67891-67903. DOI: 10.18632/oncotarget.18910

[45] Merchant AA, William M. Targeting hedgehog-a cancer stem cell pathway. Clinical Cancer Research. 2010;**16**(12):3130-3140. DOI: 10.1158/1078-0432.CCR-09-2846

[46] Lopez-Millan B, Diaz de la Guardia R, Roca-Ho H, et al. IMiDs mobilize acute myeloid leukemia blasts to peripheral blood through downregulation of CXCR4 but fail to potentiate AraC/Idarubicin activity in preclinical models of non del5q/5q- AML. OncoImmunology. 2018;**9**:e1477460. DOI: 10.1080/2162402x.2018.1477460

[47] Mulyani SWM, Ernawati DS, Astuti ER, et al. Hypoxic preconditioning effect on stromal cells derived factor-1 and C-X-C chemokine receptor type 4 expression in Wistar rat's (*Rattus norvegicus*) bone marrow mesenchymal stem cells (in vitro study). Veterinary World. 2018;**11**(7):965-970. DOI: 10.14202/vetworld.2018.965-970

[48] Kucia M, Reca R, Miekus K, et al. Trafficking of normal stem cells and metastasis of cancer stem cells involve similar mechanisms: Pivotal role of the SDF-1–CXCR4 axis. Stem Cells. 2010;**23**(7):879-894. DOI: 10.1634/stemcells.2004-0342

[49] Tsvee L, Ayelet D, Orit K. How do stem cells find their way home? Blood. 2005;**106**(6):1901-1910. DOI: 10.1182/blood-2005-04-1417

[50] Surendran S, Siddappa G, Mohan A, et al. Cancer stem cell and its niche in malignant progression of oral potentially malignant disorders. Oral Oncology. 2017;**75**:140-147. DOI: 10.1016/j.oraloncology.2017.11.003

[51] Mercurio L, Ajmone-Cat MA, Cecchetti S, et al. Targeting CXCR4 by a selective peptide antagonist modulates tumor microenvironment and microglia reactivity in a human glioblastoma model. Journal of Experimental & Clinical Cancer Research. 2016;**35**:55. DOI: 10.1186/s13046-016-0326-y

[52] Decastro AJ, Pratima C, Amanda B, et al. ΔNP63α transcriptionally activates chemokine receptor 4 (CXCR4) expression to regulate breast cancer stem cell activity and chemotaxis. Molecular Cancer Therapeutics. 2015;**14**(1):225-235. DOI: 10.1158/1535-7163.MCT-14-0194

[53] Li H, Guo L, Jie S, et al. Berberine inhibits SDF-1-induced AML cells and leukemic stem cells migration via regulation of SDF-1 level in bone marrow stromal cells. Biomedicine & Pharmacotherapy. 2008;**62**(9):573-578. DOI: 10.1016/j.biopha.2008.08.003

[54] Li H, Liu L, Guo L, et al. HERG K^+ channel expression in $CD34^+/CD38^-/$ CD123 high cells and primary leukemia cells and analysis of its regulation in leukemia cells. International Journal of Hematology. 2008;**87**(4):387-392. DOI: 10.1007/s12185-008-0056-9

[55] Mannelli F, Cutini I, Gianfaldoni G, et al. CXCR4 expression accounts for clinical phenotype and outcome in acute myeloid leukemia. Cytometry. Part B, Clinical Cytometry. 2015;**86**(5):340-349. DOI: 10.1002/cytob.21156

[56] Guo P, Gao A, Zhang G, et al. Decoding the knots of initiation of oncogenic epithelial-mesenchymal transition in tumor progression. Current Cancer Drug Targets. 2013;**13**(9):996-1011. DOI: 10.2174/15680096113136660105-

[57] Galán-Díez M, Kousteni S. The osteoblastic niche in hematopoiesis and hematological myeloid malignancies. Current Molecular Biology Reports.

2017;**3**(2):53-62. DOI: 10.1007/s40610-017-0055-9

[58] Calvi LM, Adams GB, Weibrecht KW, et al. Osteoblastic cells regulate the haematopoietic stem cell niche. Nature. 2003;**425**(6960):841-846. DOI: 10.1038/nature02040

[59] Kusumbe AP, Ramasamy SK, Itkin T, et al. Age-dependent modulation of vascular niches for haematopoietic stem cells. Nature. 2016;**532**(7599):380-384. DOI: 10.1038/nature17638

[60] Tabe Y, Konopleva M. Leukemia stem cells microenvironment. Advances in Experimental Medicine and Biology. 2017;**1041**:19-32. DOI: 10.1007/978-3-319-69194-7_3

[61] Yang JG, Wang LL, Ma DC. Effects of vascular endothelial growth factors and their receptors on megakaryocytes and platelets and related diseases. British Journal of Haematology. 2017;**180**(3):321-334. DOI: 10.1111/bjh.15000

[62] Yanfei J, Yunshan W, Jingwu X. The hedgehog pathway: Role in cell differentiation, polarity and proliferation. Archives of Toxicology. 2015;**89**(2):179-191. DOI: 10.1007/s00204-014-1433-1

[63] Fukushima N, Minami Y, Kakiuchi S, et al. Small-molecule hedgehog inhibitor attenuates the leukemia-initiation potential of acute myeloid leukemia cells. Cancer Science. 2016;**107**(10):1422-1429. DOI: 10.1111/cas.13019

[64] Long B, Wang LX, Zheng FM, et al. Targeting GLI1 suppresses cell growth and enhances chemosensitivity in CD34$^+$ enriched acute myeloid leukemia progenitor cells. Cellular Physiology and Biochemistry. 2016;**38**(4):1288-1302. DOI: 10.1159/000443075. doi, 10.1159/000443075

[65] Sadarangani A, Pineda G, Lennon KM, et al. GLI2 inhibition abrogates human leukemia stem cell dormancy. Journal of Translational Medicine. 2015;**13**:98. DOI: 10.1186/s12967-015-0453-9

[66] Teglund S, Toftgård R. Hedgehog beyond medulloblastoma and basal cell carcinoma. Biochimica et Biophysica Acta. 2010;**1805**(2):181-208. DOI: 10.1016/j.bbcan.2010.01.003

[67] Marina PDM, Matthias H. Hedgehog signalling in cancer formation and maintenance. Nature Reviews Cancer. 2003;**3**(12):903-911. DOI: 10.1038/nrc1229

[68] Yamaguchi R, Lartigue L, Perkins G. Targeting mcl-1 and other Bcl-2 family member proteins in cancer therapy. Pharmacology & Therapeutics. 2018;**pii**:S0163-7258(18)30193-1. DOI: 10.1016/j.pharmthera.2018.10.009

[69] Lin TL, Matsui W. Hedgehog pathway as a drug target: Smoothened inhibitors in development. OncoTargets and Therapy. 2012;**5**(1):47-58. DOI: 10.2147/OTT.S21957

[70] Kobune M, Takimoto R, Murase K, et al. Drug resistance is dramatically restored by hedgehog inhibitors in CD34$^+$ leukemic cells. Cancer Science. 2009;**100**(5):948-955. DOI: 10.1111/j.1349-7006.2009.01111.x

[71] Kotschy A, Szlavik Z, Murray J, et al. The MCL1 inhibitor S63845 is tolerable and effective in diverse cancer models. Nature. 2016;**538**(7626):477-482. DOI: 10.1038/nature19830

[72] Chamuleau ME, Ossenkoppele GJ, van Rhenen A, et al. High TRAIL-R3 expression on leukemic blasts is associated with poor outcome and induces apoptosis-resistance which can be overcome by targeting TRAIL-R2. Leukemia Research. 2011;**35**(6):741-749. DOI: 10.1016/j.leukres.2010.12.032

[73] Singh BN, Junsheng F, Srivastava RK, et al. Hedgehog signaling

antagonist GDC-0449 (Vismodegib) inhibits pancreatic cancer stem cell characteristics: Molecular mechanisms. PLoS One. 2011;**6**(11):e27306. DOI: 10.1371/journal.pone.0027306

[74] Li J, Volk A, Zhang J, et al. Sensitizing leukemia stem cells to NF-κB inhibitor treatment in vivo by inactivation of both TNF and IL-1 signaling. Oncotarget. 2016;**8**(5):8420-8435. DOI: 10.18632/oncotarget.14220

[75] Xu B, Wang S, Li R, et al. Disulfiram/copper selectively eradicates AML leukemia stem cells in vitro and in vivo by simultaneous induction of ROS-JNK and inhibition of NF-κB and Nrf2. Cell Death & Disease. 2017;**8**(5):e2797. DOI: 10.1038/cddis.2017.176

[76] Pei S, Minhajuddin M, D'Alessandro A, et al. Rational design of a parthenolide-based drug regimen that selectively eradicates acute myelogenous leukemia stem cells. The Journal of Biological Chemistry. 2016;**291**(42):21984-22000. DOI: 10.1074/jbc.M116.750653

[77] Ding Y, Yang Z, Ge W, et al. Synthesis and biological evaluation of dithiocarbamate esters of parthenolide as potential anti-acute myelogenous leukaemia agents. Journal of Enzyme Inhibition and Medicinal Chemistry. 2018;**33**(1):1376-1391. DOI: 10.1080/14756366.2018.1490734

[78] Liang H, Zheng QL, Fang P, et al. Targeting the PI3K/AKT pathway via GLI1 inhibition enhanced the drug sensitivity of acute myeloid leukemia cells. Scientific Reports. 2017;**7**:40361. DOI: 10.1038/srep40361

[79] Chen HP, Huang YQ, Ma XD. Antiproliferative effects of LY294002 on MCL Jeko-1 cell line and its mechanism. Zhongguo Shi Yan Xue Ye Xue Za Zhi. 2013;**21**(5):1183-1186. DOI: 10.7534/j.issn.1009-2137.2013.05.019

[80] Mise J, Dembitz V, Banfic H, et al. Combined inhibition of PI3K and mTOR exerts synergistic antiproliferative effect, but diminishes differentiative properties of rapamycin in acute myeloid leukemia cells. Pathology Oncology Research. 2011;**17**(3):645-656. DOI: 10.1007/s12253-011-9365-z

[81] Fragoso R, Barata JT. PTEN and leukemia stem cells. Advances in Biological Regulation. 2014;**56**:22-29. DOI: 10.1016/j.jbior.2014.05.005

[82] Hanahan D, Coussens L. Accessories to the crime: Functions of cells recruited to the tumor microenvironment. Cancer Cell. 2012;**21**(3):309-322. DOI: 10.1016/j.ccr.2012.02.022

[83] Passaro D, Irigoyen M, Catherinet C, et al. CXCR4 is required for leukemia-initiating cell activity in T cell acute lymphoblastic leukemia. Cancer Cell. 2015;**27**(6):769-779. DOI: 10.1016/j.ccell.2015.05.003

[84] Byung-Sik C, Zhihong Z, Hong M, et al. Antileukemia activity of the novel peptidic CXCR4 antagonist LY2510924 as monotherapy and in combination with chemotherapy. Blood. 2015;**126**(2):222-232. DOI: 10.1182/blood-2015-02-628677

[85] Becker PS, Foran JM, Altman JK, et al. Targeting the CXCR4 pathway: Safety, tolerability and clinical activity of ulocuplumab (BMS-936564), an anti-CXCR4 antibody, in relapsed/refractory acute myeloid leukemia. Blood. 2014;**124**:386

[86] Riether C, Schürch CM, Ochsenbein AF. Regulation of hematopoietic and leukemic stem cells by the immune system. Cell Death and Differentiation. 2015;**22**(2):187-198. DOI: 10.1038/cdd.2014.89

[87] Fujisaki J, Wu J, Carlson AL, et al. In vivo imaging of treg cells providing immune privilege to the

haematopoietic stem-cell niche. Nature. 2011;**474**(7350):216-219. DOI: 10.1038/nature10160

[88] Celalettin U, Miller JS, Munn DH, et al. Regulatory T cells in acute myelogenous leukemia: Is it time for immunomodulation? Blood. 2011;**118**(19):5084-5095. DOI: 10.1182/blood-2011-07-365817

[89] Lane SW, Scadden DT, Gilliland DG. The leukemic stem cell niche: Current concepts and therapeutic opportunities. Blood. 2009;**114**(6):1150-1157. DOI: 10.1182/blood-2009-01-202606

[90] Carsten R, Schürch CM, Christoph F, et al. Tyrosine kinase inhibitor-induced CD70 expression mediates drug resistance in leukemia stem cells by activating Wnt signaling. Science Translational Medicine. 2015;7(298):298ra119. DOI: 10.1126/scitranslmed.aab1740

[91] Min C, Paolo G, Donna DG, et al. Targeting primitive chronic myeloid leukemia cells by effective inhibition of a new AHI-1-BCR-ABL-JAK2 complex. Journal of the National Cancer Institute. 2013;**105**(6):405-423. DOI: 10.1093/jnci/djt006

[92] Lin XC, Liu XG, Zhang YM, et al. Integrated analysis of microRNA and transcription factor reveals important regulators and regulatory motifs in adult B-cell acute lymphoblastic leukemia. International Journal of Oncology. 2017;**50**(2):671-683. DOI: 10.3892/ijo.2016.3832

[93] Annesley CE, Brown P. The biology and targeting of FLT3 in pediatric leukemia. Frontiers in Oncology. 2014;**4**:263. DOI: 10.3389/fonc.2014.00263

[94] Ruth S, Andrea HK, Florian B, et al. CDK6 as a key regulator of hematopoietic and leukemic stem cell activation. Blood. 2015;**125**(1):90-101. DOI: 10.1182/blood-2014-06-584417

[95] Appelbaum FR, Bernstein ID. Gemtuzumab ozogamicin for acute myeloid leukemia. Blood. 2017;**130**(22):2373-2376. DOI: 10.1182/blood-2017-09-797712

[96] Dutour A, Marin V, Pizzitola I, et al. In vitro and in vivo antitumor effect of anti-CD33 chimeric receptor-expressing EBV-CTL against CD33 acute myeloid leukemia. Advances in Hematology. 2012;**2012**:683065. DOI: 10.1155/2012/683065

[97] Ho TC, LaMere M, Stevens BM, et al. Evolution of acute myelogenous leukemia stem cell properties after treatment and progression. Blood. 2016;**128**(13):1671-1678. DOI: 10.1182/blood-2016-02-695312

Chapter 3

Pediatric Acute Lymphoblastic Leukemia: Recent Advances for a Promising Future

Sneha Tandon and Angela S. Punnett

Abstract

Acute lymphoblastic leukemia (ALL) is the most common pediatric cancer and accounts for approximately 75% of all cases of childhood leukemia. Both diagnostic and therapeutic advances have been instrumental in improving the outcomes of once a dreaded disease. Currently, approximately 90% of the children treated according to risk-directed and response-adapted therapy will be long-term survivors. The use of pediatric protocols for the treatment of adolescent and young adults (AYA) has also resulted in significant improvements in their long-term survival. New therapies including tyrosine kinase inhibitors (TKIs), monoclonal antibodies and CAR T-cell therapy are changing the approach to therapy for relapsed or refractory disease. We are approaching a time where therapy for all patients will be personalized with the use of genome-based characterization of disease and incorporation of drugs against actionable targets, ultimately leading to improved clinical outcomes and decreased toxicity of therapy. Still, certain subgroups including patients with relapsed disease, infant ALL, and those with certain cytogenetic/molecular variants, remain challenging to treat. This chapter is an overview of the recent advances in the ALL disease biology, newly identified prognostic factors and an overview of emerging therapeutic options.

Keywords: acute lymphoblastic leukemia, minimal residual disease, CAR T-cell therapy, monoclonal antibody, advances

1. Background

ALL is the most common childhood malignancy and accounts for approximately 30% of all childhood cancers and 75% of all cases of childhood leukemia [1, 2]. Each year, 3600 new cases of childhood ALL are diagnosed in the United States. Precursor B-ALL accounts for approximately 80–85% of the cases, while 15–20% are of the T-cell type [3]. The peak age group for ALL is 2–8 years, which accounts for approximately 80% of the childhood ALL burden. The incidence decreases from 90 cases per million in the 2-8-year age group to 30 per million beyond 8 years of age [3, 4]. ALL is more common in children compared to older age groups as shown in **Figures 1** and **2** [5].

The treatment of childhood ALL has evolved over the past 50 years. Successful development of multi-agent chemotherapy regimens, improved disease risk stratification as well as enhanced supportive care have been instrumental in improving survival (**Figure 3**) [6]. The ALL chemotherapy backbone has included various phases—remission induction, central nervous system-directed therapy, interim maintenance and continuation therapy—with essentially the same chemotherapy

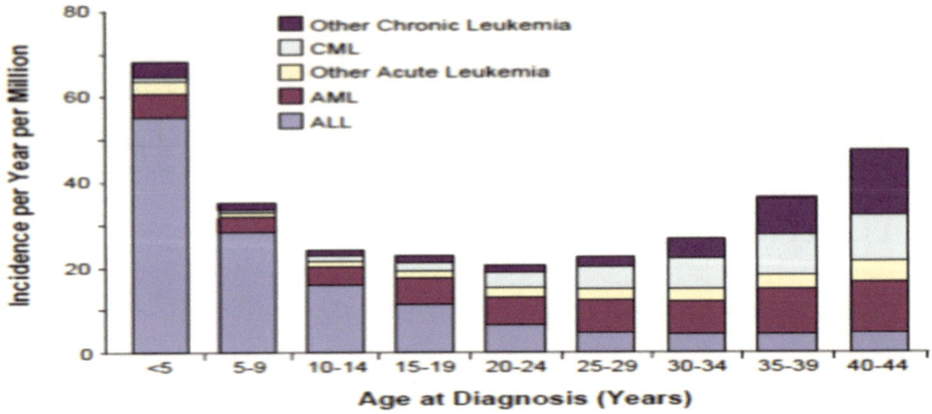

Figure 1.
Incidence of leukemia by age, SEER 1975–1999 [6].

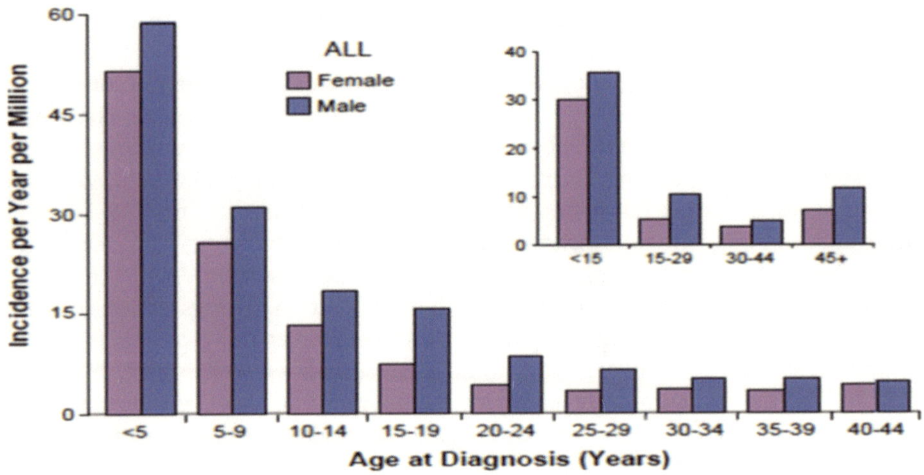

Figure 2.
Incidence of acute lymphoblastic leukemia by age and gender, SEER, 1975–1999 [6].

drugs in use since the 1960s. Modifications in dosing, mode of administration and varying combinations have resulted in improvements in outcomes now reaching a plateau [7–10]. Certain subgroups continue to have a very poor outcome, including those patients with relapsed disease, infant ALL, and specific disease-related cytogenetic and molecular changes.

Childhood ALL differs from adult ALL in several ways. The overall survival (OS) of pediatric ALL has reached 90%, whereas adults still fare poorly at approximately 40% [10, 11]. Biologically, there is a higher frequency of poor prognostic subtypes like Philadelphia (Ph) positive and multi-lineage leukemia (MLL) rearranged leukemia in adults compared to children (7% vs. 1–2%) [12]. On the contrary, children have a higher frequency of favorable cytogenetics like hyperdiploidy and ETV6-RUNX1 as their leukemia drivers [12]. The majority of children with ALL are treated at specialized centres and as part of clinical trials, unlike adults. Additionally, pediatric protocols have a greater dose intensity and deliver therapy guided by degree of myelosuppression. Adults generally tolerate treatment less well, resulting in increased treatment related toxicity

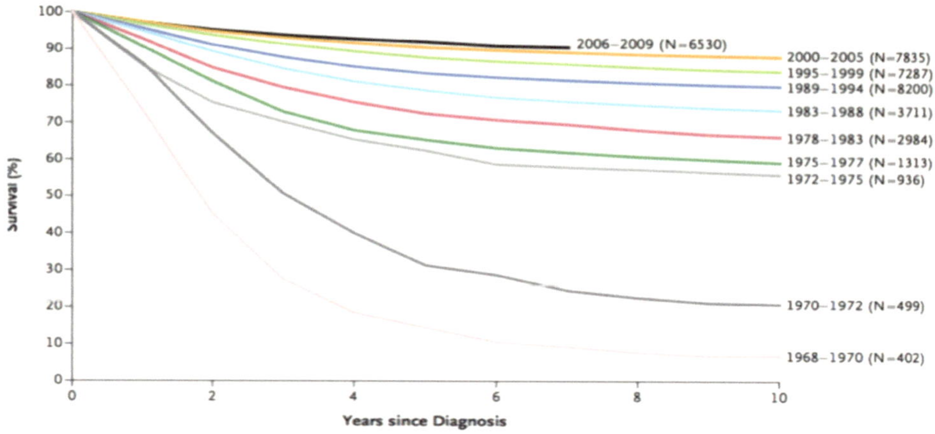

Figure 3.
Overall survival of children with acute lymphoblastic leukemia who were treated in the Children's Cancer Group and Children's Oncology Group trials between 1968 and 2009 (reprinted from Ref. [6], Copyright (2015) with permission from Massachusetts Medical Society).

[13]. The increased treatment related toxicity in adults could also be due to the increased use of stem cell transplant (SCT) in first remission, unlike the pediatric population where it is reserved only for high risk, poor responding or relapsed subgroups. Additionally, the use of pediatric-type protocols for the treatment of adolescent and young adults has resulted in significant improvements in their long-term survival [14, 15].

2. Minimal residual disease (MRD)-guided therapy

Minimal residual disease measured post-induction has been shown to be most predictive of long-term outcomes across various studies [16–18]. It is an amalgam of leukemia biology, patient factors as well as therapy. With the current protocol-based, risk-directed therapy complemented by MRD based risk stratification, approximately 90% of the children aged 1–18 years are expected to be long-term survivors [19–22]. Various sensitive techniques have been utilized for evaluation of MRD including multi-color flow-cytometry (MFC), RT-PCR and next generation sequencing, which can detect 1 leukemic cell in 10,000–100,000 normal cells [16]. Analysis and tracking of Ig/TCR gene rearrangements by PCR is feasible in 90% of B and T-ALL and detection of fusion gene transcripts in approximately 30–40%. Other new techniques of MRD analysis include high-throughput sequencing (HTS) of Ig/TCR with a sensitivity of 1 in 1 million cells (10^{-6}) [23]. In a recent study by Wood et al., HTS and MFC were comparable and HTS produced similar results as regards the prognostic significance of MRD [23]. Therapy modification based on MRD in the UKALL2003 and the Dutch ALL10 trial was associated with improved outcomes in childhood ALL [22, 24]. The AIEOP-BFM-ALL 2000 trial showed improved outcomes in both pediatric B and T ALL with MRD based therapy [25]. With the use of clinical and biological factors to stratify children with ALL into various risk groups, risk-directed therapy has led to the delivery of less intense as well as less toxic therapy to the low risk groups and more intensive therapy to those with a higher probability of relapse and poorer outcomes.

Despite high cure rates for pediatric ALL, up to 20% of the children will relapse. Re-induction for this group of patients yields remission in 79–90% of patients, however long-term survival is only 40–50% [26, 27]. Moreover, the outcomes are worse in patients with primary refractory or relapse and refractory disease (r/r) as well as relapse post SCT; hence the unmet need for durable therapies for such children. The incorporation of newer therapies including monoclonal antibodies and Chimeric Antigen Receptor (CAR) T-cell therapy offer an alternative approach to the management of relapsed/refractory pediatric B ALL. The increasing use of upfront genome-based characterization of disease, and incorporation of drugs against identified actionable targets, will ultimately lead to improved clinical outcomes and deceased toxicity of therapy. This chapter will focus on the recent diagnostic and therapeutic advances which are changing the way children with ALL are treated.

3. Novel diagnostics in ALL

The recent WHO 2016 classification has incorporated morphological, immunophenotypic and the existing cytogenetic features with the new molecular features associated with the various subgroups of ALL [28]. Cytogenetic/molecular abnormalities have been identified in 60–80% of patients with ALL using traditional methods [29]; however, with the advent of genome-wide analysis, this number is expected to increase. Evolution of the diagnostics from morphology, immunohistochemistry, and banding techniques to genome-wide analysis and epigenomics has led to an increased appreciation of the biology of leukemia. Genome-wide studies have also provided insight into the variation in the response to chemotherapy drugs among patients, explaining both the differences in toxicities and response to therapy [30]. In the near future, it can be envisioned that ALL will be molecularly characterized and defined, thus enabling us to deliver tailored therapy.

4. Existing and novel genomics of ALL

Cytogenetic aberrations in ALL have emerged as one of the most important prognostic factors driving the biology of the disease and patient outcomes [29]. Existing and recently identified novel prognostic markers are illustrated in **Figure 4** [31]. Children carrying either high hyperdiploidy (51–65 chromosomes) or ETV6-RUNX1 as their cytogenetic drivers have an excellent prognosis with survival of >90% at 5 years. Adverse prognostic factors include t(9; 22), MLL translocation, t(17; 19), complex karyotype, low hypodiploidy (31–39 chromosomes), near haploidy (24–30 chromosomes), and near triploidy (60–78 chromosomes) [13]. Germline TP53 mutations are seen in children with ALL and low hypodiploidy (chromosomes 31–39) and confer a poor prognosis [32]. New additions to the list of adverse prognostic factors include BCR-ABL-1 like mutations, iAMP21, CRFL2 overexpression, JAK mutations, and translocations involving immunoglobulin heavy chain (IGH), TCF-PBX1, IKZF1, PAX5, ERG and EBF1 mutations [31, 33–37]. Association of CDKN2A/2B deletions with Ph + ALL have emerged as a poor prognostic factor with guarded prognosis even with SCT [33]. FLT3 mutations have been found in KMT2A rearranged infant ALL and confer a poor prognosis [38–40]. Growing understanding of the biology of the disease allows better risk stratification and in some cases alterations to therapy to improve outcomes. For example, therapy intensification has resulted in improved outcomes in children harboring the iAMP21 mutation [41, 42].

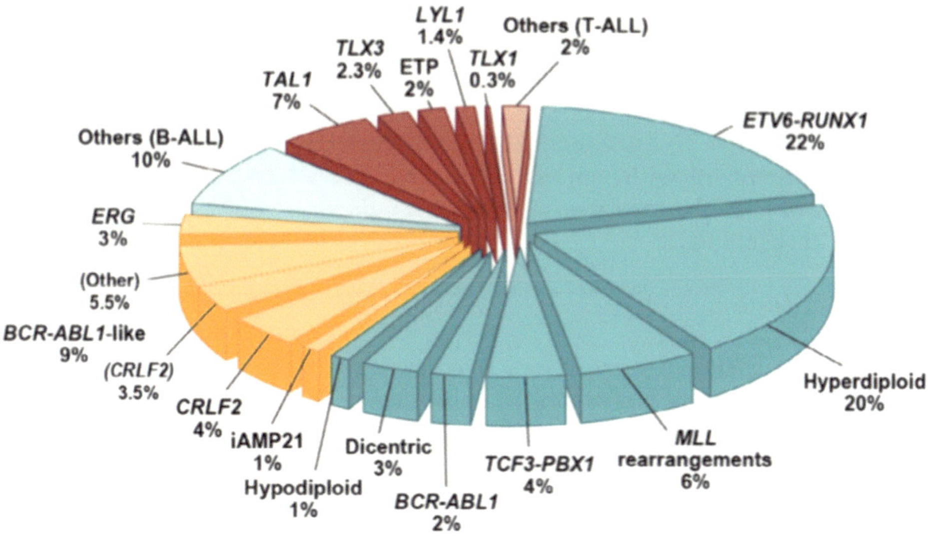

Figure 4.
Sub-classification of childhood ALL. Blue wedges refer to B-progenitor ALL, yellow to recently identified subtypes of B-ALL, and red wedges to T-lineage ALL (reprinted from Ref. [31], copyright (2013) with permission from Elsevier).

In T-cell ALL, mutations commonly found are those involved in T-cell development. Mutations of the NOTCH-1 activating gene are seen in approximately 50–60% of all the T-ALL cases, while mutations involving the tumor suppressor gene FBXW7 are found in approximately 15% of cases [43]. The French group (FRALLE) has demonstrated favorable outcomes in those with NOTCH/FBXW7 mutations along with wild-type PTEN/RAS [44]. However, the prognostic significance of these in T-ALL is not well defined [45, 46]. Genome-wide association studies have recently identified a number of inherited genetic polymorphisms that are associated with an increased predisposition to develop ALL. These novel genes include ARID5B, GATA3, IKZF1, CDKN2A, CDKN2B, PIP4K2A and TP63 [47–53].

4.1 Novel genomics

Salient features of the novel prognostic factors are described below:

4.1.1 Ph-like ALL

BCR-ABL1-like ALL has recently been recognized by sequencing studies by the COG-St Jude consortium (TARGET) and the DCOG, and disease shows a similar gene expression profile to that of Ph + ALL in the absence of the BCR-ABL-1 gene translocation [54–56]. This accounts for 10% of pediatric and 15–20% of AYA ALL and confers an extremely poor prognosis with 5-year disease free survival (DFS) of 25% in AYA patients [34, 54]. The AALL0331 study showed decrease prevalence of Ph-like ALL in children with NCI standard risk (SR) compared to high risk (HR) ALL [57]. Ph-like ALL harbors two types of genomic alterations namely *kinase activating* and *cytokine receptor alterations* [58]. The kinase alterations which can be inhibited by ABL inhibitors include *ABL1*, *ABL2*, colony stimulating factor 1 receptor (*CSF1R*), platelet-derived growth factor receptor alfa and beta (*PDGFRA*, *PDGFRB*) [34]. Cytokine receptor alterations include alterations that act via the *JAK/STAT* pathway. This includes membrane-bound thymic stromal lymphopoietin receptor *(TSLRP)/CRLF2*. Other pathways involving CRLF2 include *PI3K* and the *mTOR* pathways [58]. *CRLF2* gene rearrangements have been associated with 50% of the cases of Ph-like ALL, of which another 50% also show positivity for *JAK* mutations [33, 56]. Additionally, *IKZF1*deletions (28%), *EPOR, RAS* pathway (10%) are also seen in this group. Patients harboring the *CRLF2* alterations fare poorly with high risk of relapse [59]. Similarly, increased expression of *IKZF1* possibly translates into high post induction MRD as well as higher risk of relapse [60, 61].

4.1.2 IKZF1 deletions

The *IKZF1* deletion has recently emerged as a novel genomic marker in childhood ALL. This subtype is commonly seen in older children, those with higher WBC counts, Down syndrome (DS), BCR-ABL and Ph-like ALL [55, 59, 62, 63]. Increased association is also seen with *CRLF2* mutations [62]. *IKZF1* deletion is an independent poor prognostic genomic feature in multivariate analysis [64–68]. The AIEOP-BFM group showed *IKZF1* deletions confer a poor prognosis only in the high end-induction MRD group with co-existent *CDKN2A*, *CDKN2B*, *PAX5*, or *PAR1* mutations [69].

4.1.3 JAK-pathway mutations.

JAK mutations are commonly found in Ph-like ALL (20%) and are also associated with *CRLF2* mutations [33]. These are also seen in approximately 15% of children with DS ALL [34, 70, 71]. Identification of this mutation is essential as it has therapeutic implications with responses seen both *in vitro and in vivo* to TKIs [72]. The ongoing phase II trial AALL1521 is testing upfront addition of ruxolitinib to chemotherapy for *CRFL2* rearranged or *JAK*-pathway mutant children with ALL [73].

4.1.4 Immunoglobulin heavy chain gene (IGH) rearrangement, CRLF2 overexpression

IGH, a novel, adverse prognostic, cytogenetic driver is seen in less than 3% of pediatric and 10% of AYA ALL [74]. This rearrangement is characterized by the juxtaposition of a partner oncogene like *CRLF2* (25%) or *CEBP* (10%) with *IGH* that drives the overexpression. *CRLF2* overexpression is seen in a very high proportion (>50%) of children with DS, but the prognostic significance is still unclear [59].

4.1.5 iAMP21

This novel prognostic marker is seen in about 1.5–2% of pediatric ALL and is characterized by ≥3 extra copies of *RUNX1* gene on a single abnormal chromosome 21q22 [75, 76]. Increased predisposition to develop *iAMP21* ALL is seen in carriers of the Robertsonian translocation involving chromosomes 15 and 21 [77]. This subtype presents in older children (median 10 years), is more common in females, and presents with WBC count of less than 50×10^9/L. Presence of this mutation confers a poor prognosis with standard therapy as well as high post remission-induction MRD [41, 78, 79]. However, the outcomes are better with MRD-guided and intensive chemotherapy, as shown in the UKALL2003 and the ALL-BFM 2000 studies, hence precluding the need for SCT in first remission [41, 42].

4.2 Treatment

4.2.1 Adolescents and young adults (AYA) with ALL

AYA constitutes a unique group of ALL with an age range of 15–39 years as defined by the NCI. Based on disease biology, there has always been a debate as to the best regimen to be used in this age group. Historically, ALL in the AYA population has been associated with a poor outcome and higher treatment related morbidity. However, the current focus of treating AYA as per pediatric protocols has resulted in improvement in their outcomes [14, 15] as shown in **Table 1**. Chemotherapy protocols similar to the BFM backbone with corticosteroids, vincristine and asparaginase in induction, post-remission asparaginase, and CNS prophylaxis during induction have shown improved survival in this cohort of patients. Also, SCT is offered only to the very-high risk population in first complete remission (CR1) [80].

To support this further, the excellent results from the large study by the GRAALL group have shown significantly improved survival (66% vs. 44%, $P < 0.001$) for those treated with pediatric-inspired protocols compared to historical controls treated with adult protocols [81]. The largest study which has evaluated this hypothesis is the US intergroup trial C10403, in which 318 AYA patients were treated as per the standard arm of the COG AALL0232 protocol. Encouraging results from this study showed a 2-year event free survival (EFS) of 66% and overall survival (OS) of 78%, with manageable toxicity profile and subsequently the NCI recommended that pediatric-inspired protocols could be used effectively up to the age of 40 years [82].

4.2.2 Philadelphia-chromosome positive ALL (Ph + ALL)

This high-risk group of ALL constitutes about 20–30% of the adult ALL and 3% of pediatric ALL [88]. Approximately 90% of the pediatric Ph + ALL have the p190 translocation, which results from the translocation within the 'minor' breakpoint cluster region (mBCR) [89]. It is also characterized by a high frequency (66%) of deletions in B-cell development genes like IKZF1, PAX5, EBF1 and CDKN2A/B. [33, 88, 90]. Historically, outcomes were extremely poor with 5-year OS of 19%

Serial no.	Study group	Patients numbers (n)	Median age (y)	Survival (%)
1.	CCG [14]	197	16	67, OS 7y
2.	CALGB [15]	124	19	46
3.	FRALLE93 [15]	77	16	67 EFS
4.	AIEOP [83, 84]	150	15	80, OS 2y
5.	DCOG [85]	47	12	71 EFS
6.	NOPHO92 [86]	36	16	74, OS 5y
7.	MRC ALL [87]	61	15–17	71, OS 5y
8.	UKALL2003 [24]	229	16–24	72 EFS

CCG, Children's Cancer Group; CALGB, Cancer and Leukemia Group; FRALLE, French Acute lymphoblastic Leukemia Study Group; AIEOP, Associazione Italiana di Ematologia e Oncologia Pediatrica; DCOG, Dutch Childhood Oncology Group; NOPHO, Nordic Society for Pediatric Hematology and Oncology; MRC ALL, Medical Research Council (United Kingdom).

Table 1.
Improved outcomes for AYA when treated according to pediatric-based protocols.

without transplant and 35–45% with transplant in CR1. However, survival has drastically improved with the advent of TKIs as seen in the UKALLXII/ECOG2993 study, 4-year OS with imatinib compared to historical cohort, 38% vs. 22% [91]. The AALL0031 reported excellent 5-year EFS of 70% ± 12% in patients treated with continuous imatinib and intensive chemotherapy compared with 31–39% for historical controls [92, 93]. Second generation TKIs are highly potent, demonstrate faster and deeper remissions, as well as increased CNS activity with an acceptable toxicity profile. The COG AALL0622 trial, did not show any survival advantage of dasatinib over imatinib when added to upfront chemotherapy backbone, 5-year OS 81% vs. 86% for AALL0031 and AALL0622 respectively. In the same study, IKZF1 deletions were identified in 57% of cases and were associated with inferior outcomes [94].

Ph + ALL is no longer considered a subgroup for allogeneic SCT in CR1, and is reserved for poor responders or for relapsed disease. The AALL0031 study showed improved 3-year EFS equal to or better than sibling-related SCT (88% vs. 57%) for patients treated with imatinib and intensive systemic chemotherapy. Long-term follow-up data from the same study showed 5-year DFS of 70% in the imatinib plus chemotherapy group compared to SCT (65%-sibling donor, 59%-unrelated donor) [93]. The Korean Society of Adult Hematology working party showed similar 2-year molecular relapse-free survival in those not transplanted versus those transplanted (65% vs. 53%) [95]. In a study by Ravandi et al., achievement of negative MRD status was a significant prognostic factor regulating long-term survival. The 4-year OS rates were 66, 43 and 32% in patients with 3-month CMR, major molecular remission (MMR) and less than MMR, respectively [96]. Hence, adequate molecular response is the deciding factor for no SCT versus SCT.

With regards to the use of TKIs in the post-transplantation period, the consensus statement of the Acute Leukemia Working Party of the European Society for Blood and Marrow Transplantation, recommends patients with undetectable MRD post allogenic SCT may be either treated prophylactically or, may be monitored and treated pre-emptively with TKI if they have detectable MRD post-transplant. TKIs may be continued for a period of 12 months of continuous MRD negativity for those undergoing SCT in CR1, and continued indefinitely for those undergoing SCT in ≥2nd CR status [97]. Currently AALL1631, an international collaborative trial between the COG and the EsPhALL groups, is testing combination chemotherapy with imatinib in Ph + ALL. This randomized trial will assess survival and toxicity outcomes with less intensive therapy for those who are MRD negative post induction compared to the current EsPhALL and COG AALL1122 protocols. The role of post-transplant imatinib in the high-risk group of Ph + ALL undergoing SCT is also being evaluated [98].

4.2.3 Philadelphia-like ALL (Ph-like ALL)

Ph-like ALL constitutes a high-risk subtype of pediatric B ALL. Most studies demonstrate a poorer prognosis despite augmented traditional chemotherapy [54, 57, 70]. Interestingly, the Total XV study showed MRD directed therapy negated its poor prognosis [99]. Research is currently ongoing for a better understanding of the genomics of this group and we now know that this group harbors certain targetable genetic alterations. Potential targets and agents tested in preclinical models include; *CRLF2* inhibition (Givinostat [100], Luminespib [101], Selumetinib [102], TSLPR CART cells [103]), *JAK-2* (CHZ868) [104], *mTOR* pathway (Rapamycin) [105], *PI3K* and *mTOR* pathways (Gedatolisib) [106], and *TNF-a* inhibition (Birinapant) [107]. These targets are now being prospectively studies in clinical trials across various centres. The MDACC trial in children older than 10 years is testing ruxolitinib or dasatinib with chemotherapy [108].

Also, the phase II COG AALL1521 study is testing ruxolitinib with conventional chemotherapy in the age group of 1–21 years [109]. Another phase II trial from the NCI (COG AALL1131) in 1–30-year olds is testing dasatinib in combination with chemotherapy [110].

4.2.4 Hypodiploid ALL

Hypodiploidy (<45 chromosomes) is present in less than 5% of ALL. Survival across various studies ranges between 50 and 60% on currently available therapy [111–113]. Near haploid (24–30 chromosomes) and low-hypodiploidy (chromosome 31–39) fare poorly on current protocols with 5–8-year EFS of 25–40% for near-haploid and 30–50% for low-hypodiploid ALL [111, 112, 114]. Interestingly, MRD has emerged as an important prognostic marker; improved long-term survival is seen in those with MRD negativity post induction compared to MRD positive disease as shown by Mullighan et al. (85.1% vs. 44.4%) [115]. Recent studies show that children carrying pathogenic germline TP53 mutations have a significantly higher incidence of hypodiploidy (65% vs. 1%), inferior EFS, OS and a very high chance of developing second cancers [92]. Also, a significantly large proportion (91.2%) of low hypodiploidy ALL is associated with germline TP53 mutation suggesting a possible association of hypodiploid ALL with Li-Fraumeni syndrome. In a study by Holmfeldt et al., near-haploid ALL was found to be associated with *RAS*-signaling, *CREBBP*, *CDKN2A/B*, *PAG1* and *IKZF3*, and low hypodiploidy with *P53*, *IKZF2*, *RB1*, *histone modifiers* and *CDKN2A/B* [32, 116, 117]. The COG ALL03B1 showed no survival benefit from CR1 SCT. Interestingly, this was also true if children were MRD (>0.01%) positive pre-transplant [113]. Novel therapeutic approaches with emphasis on molecular targets could be the way forward in improving the outcomes of this high-risk subset of pediatric ALL.

4.2.5 Down syndrome ALL

Children with Down syndrome (DS) have an increased predisposition compared to non-DS children to develop ALL with a cumulative risk of approximately 2.1% by age of 5 years and 2.7% by age of 30 [118, 119]. Children with DS constitute a very special group of pediatric ALL characterized by predominantly B immunophenotype and a marked absence of T immunophenotype. This group is neither associated with the favorable nor the unfavorable cytogenetic abnormalities as seen in common pediatric ALL [120]. *IKZF1* gene deletion, seen in approximately 35% of DS ALL portends inferior outcome [121, 122]. About 50–60% of the children with DS ALL harbor *CRLF2* mutation, much higher than in children with ALL without DS (<10%). Approximately, 20% of children with DS ALL also carry *JAK2* mutations, with majority also harboring *CRLF2* mutation. However, their prognostic significance is unknown [121, 123, 124].

4.2.6 Infant ALL

This rare group comprises 2–4% of pediatric ALL and is characterized by high leukocyte count at diagnosis, bulky extramedullary disease, frequent CNS involvement, and a poor prognosis [125, 126]. A relatively large proportion of these infants harbor the KMT2A gene on chromosome 11q23 in their malignant clone. [127, 128]. To date, approximately 94 different partner genes of KMT2A have been identified, with AF4 being the commonest [129]. These leukemia may contain FLT3 mutations (18%) and are characterized by overexpression of homeobox

(HOX) genes [130–133]. Younger age is associated with worse outcome. Despite intensified therapy across various trials groups including COG and Interfant, the 5-year EFS remains poor (34–37%) in the KMT2A-rearranged infants [127, 128, 134]. The role of SCT in CR1 remains controversial. Japanese and COG P9407 studies have not shown any survival benefit with SCT compared to standard chemotherapy alone [134, 135]. The COG study AALL0631 failed to demonstrate any survival benefit with the upfront addition of lestaurtinib to the chemotherapy backbone, despite high levels of FLT3 expression [39, 136]. The COG pilot study AALL15P1, is evaluating the role of upfront addition of azacytidine in combination with standard chemotherapy (Interfant protocol) for epigenetic modification in KMT2A rearranged infant ALL [137].

4.2.7 T ALL

The outcomes for T ALL have been historically very poor, however with current therapeutic approaches, outcomes are now comparable to those of B ALL with 5-year EFS of 85% [138, 139]. MRD has emerged as the most important prognostic factor. Interestingly, kinetics of MRD clearance in T-ALL is slower than B-ALL, with late MRD negativity post-consolidation still translating into improved outcomes (7-year EFS, 80.6% ± 2.3%) [140]. The UKALL2003 and the AIEOP-BFM 2000 trials have shown decreased relapse risk and survival benefit with the use of dexamethasone [138, 140]. Currently, the COG AALL1231 randomized trial is evaluating the role of bortezomib during induction and delayed intensification in patients with newly diagnosed T-cell ALL in the age group of 1–30 years using an augmented BFM-like backbone. Interestingly, this trial is also testing dexamethasone vs. prednisolone during induction and the benefit of the addition of asparaginase during maintenance therapy. Increasingly, cooperative groups are moving away from the use of prophylactic cranial radiation or restricting its use to high risk disease or CNS 3 status in upfront therapy [10, 11, 138, 141, 142]. The COG AALL1231 randomized trial is currently testing the safety of omitting prophylactic cranial irradiation in the non-high risk and non-CNS3 cases. The recent pilot AALL00P2 study tested upfront incorporation of nelarabine in newly diagnosed T ALL and has shown improved 5-year EFS of 73% for all patients and 69% for those with slow early response [143]. The COG AALL0434 randomized study tested nelarabine in frontline therapy and demonstrated safety, however final results are awaited [144]. Allogenic SCT is currently reserved only for those with positive MRD post consolidation [145].

Relapse T-ALL still remains a therapeutic challenge as the salvage rates and OS are less than 25%. In the AALL01P2 study, out of 7 patients with relapsed T-ALL, only 2 achieved CR2 [146]. However, encouraging results from the AALL07P1 trial have shown CR2 of 68% by the addition of bortezomib to a 4-drug re-induction regimen [147]. The focus is on optimizing upfront therapy to prevent relapse in the high-risk patients, with increasing efforts directed at developing effective salvage therapies for relapsed disease. Genomic sequencing studies have identified mutations related to various signaling pathways like *JAK/STAT*, *NOTCH*, *PI3K/Akt/mTOR* and *MAPK* with emerging pre-clinical evidence for targeted therapy [116, 148, 149]. Pre-clinical studies are also underway for the development of CD5 directed CAR T-cell therapy [117] as well as NK cell CARs against the T-ALL (personal communication from DiPersio and Rezvani).

4.2.8 Early T-precursor (ETP) ALL

ETP ALL has emerged as a new entity with increased heterogeneity at the molecular level. This subtype harbors *NOTCH1* mutation at a much lower frequency than T-ALL. It has a transcriptional profile similar to normal hematopoietic and myeloid stem cells [150]. Comparative genomic hybridization studies have shown absence of biallelic deletion of the TCR gamma locus (ABGD) and inferior outcomes with early treatment failure in this sub-group. [151, 152]. Other pathways implicated are the *JAK/STAT*, *PI3K/Akt/mTOR*, *FLT3*, and *MAPK* [153, 154]. Ruxolitinib, a *JAK1/2* inhibitor has shown single-agent activity in pre-clinical studies [155]. There is emerging evidence that treatment on high risk regimens and MRD guided therapy leads to similar outcomes to those of standard T ALL [156, 157].

4.2.9 Immune-targeting in relapsed/refractory B-ALL

4.2.10 Role of monoclonal antibodies in paediatric ALL

The role of monoclonal antibodies against human differentiation antigens was first demonstrated by Kohler and Milstein using hybridomas with a goal of treatment of hematological malignancies [158]. ALL is an excellent candidate for the incorporation of monoclonal antibody therapy due to a fairly constant lineage-specific antigen expression on the blasts and minimal expression of target antigen on normal tissues. Studies have demonstrated high remission rates with these agents, non-overlapping and manageable toxicity profiles leading to the FDA approval of these treatments for pediatric ALL. Monoclonal antibodies like blinatumomab and inotuzumab ozogamicin (InO) have shown excellent remission rates in pediatric ALL. The COG is currently evaluating antibodies like alemtuzumab, rituximab, blinatumomab, InO, and epratuzumab, both in r/r ALL as well as in newly diagnosed B-ALL in combination with standard chemotherapy, with a potential in future to be either incorporated with upfront therapy or replace certain components of standard of care chemotherapy.

4.2.11 Blinatumomab

Blinatumomab is a bi-specific T-cell engager antibody with binding sites to CD19 on B cells and to CD3 on T cells. Binding activates cytotoxic T cells, which induce cell death in the leukemic cell via the perforin system [159]. This drug is administered as a continuous infusion over 28 days and has shown acceptable activity and safety in various trials and was first FDA approved in December, 2014 for use in r/r Ph negative ALL. Pioneering work by Topp et al. in a phase II, single-arm clinical trial showed that 80 % (16 of 20) of MRD positive patients became MRD negative post first cycle of blinatumomab [160]. Encouraging results from the BLAST trial, wherein 78% of the MRD positive patients became negative post one cycle of blinatumomab led to its FDA approval in MRD positive settings as well [161].

In a phase I/II trial in 70 children <18 years of age with r/r ALL who were treated with single agent blinatumomab, 39% (27) achieved CR and MRD negativity in 52% [162, 163]. The AALL1331 phase III randomized trial is testing whether upfront addition of blinatumomab improves DFS in first relapse of ALL. In this trial all patients receive UK ALL R3 protocol for remission induction. Subsequently, the low risk group gets randomized to either control arm of R3 protocol or to receive three cycles of blinatumomab along with chemotherapy. The intermediate and the high-risk groups are randomized to either chemotherapy or two cycles of blinatumomab along with chemotherapy before proceeding to SCT. This trial is currently accruing patients and the results are awaited [164].

4.2.12 Inotuzumab ozogamicin (InO)

InO is a monoclonal antibody against CD22 and conjugated to calicheamicin, a potent cytotoxic compound which binds to the DNA in the leukemic blasts, resulting in double-stranded DNA breaks and cell death via apoptosis [165]. It was FDA approved in August, 2017 for use in r/r ALL. In a phase II study in r/r ALL in the age group of 6–80 years, Kantarijian et al. demonstrated ORR of 57% with median OS of 6.7 months [166]. In phase III INO-VATE trial in relapsed adult B ALL, single agent InO showed superior outcome compared to standard chemotherapy with CR (81%) and 1-year OS (78%) [167] However, its use in pediatric population continues in development. A retrospective French study in children <18 years with r/r B-ALL showed promising results (CR 72%), with hepatic and hematologic toxicities [168]. Bhojwani et al. in r/r pediatric ALL showed high CR rate (67%) with MRD negativity, independent of cytogenetic subtype or prior lines of therapy [169]. The AALL1621 phase II randomized trial in the age group 1-21 years is evaluating the role of InO in children and young adults with r/r CD22+ B ALL [170].

4.2.13 CAR T-cell therapy: the new driving force for relapsed ALL

Relapsed or refractory ALL is one of the leading causes of childhood cancer mortality. Refractory ALL in particular has a dismal prognosis with significant chemotherapy resistance in the leukemic clone. The advent of CAR T-cell therapy has brought a paradigm shift in the management of children with highly resistant disease. Rosenberg et al. at the NCI pioneered the CAR T-cell therapy and demonstrated successful treatment of cancer using CAR T-cells. This attractive therapy harnesses the immune system of the host to eradicate the leukemic clone. Adoptive T-cell therapy involves engineering T-cell receptors (TCRs) to bind to specific antigens present on tumor cells. These modified TCRs, known as CARs, allow the immune system to specifically target and destroy tumor cells in an MHC independent manner, bypassing the immune escape mechanisms of downregulation of MHC class I antigens and altered antigen processing by tumor cells [171]. These modified T cells have the capacity to expand and proliferate in the host, produce cytokines to kill tumor cells, as well as cross blood-brain barrier as shown by Maude et al. [172].

Early results from ongoing trials have shown promising and durable responses. Current complete remission rate of 90% have been reported as per the CHP959 phase I study [172]. The ELIANA [173] and ENSIGN [174] trials in r/r B ALL showed high CR rates of 90%, significantly higher than salvage rates of 30% attained with chemotherapy [26, 175]. This led to the FDA approval of CD19 4-1BB CAR T-cell therapy in August 2017 for children and young adults up to the age of 25 years. Maude et al. showed durable remission and survival in children treated with CD19 CAR T cell therapy with EFS (50%) and OS (76%) at 12 months of follow-up [176]. Success from pediatric CAR T-cell therapy trials is driving research programs across ages and disease types worldwide. The advantage of this therapy is that it can be offered to patients who are ineligible for transplant or have relapsed post-transplant, with a potential to ultimately replace SCT.

Tumor lysis syndrome, cytokine release syndrome and neurotoxicity are known complications of this therapy [177]. Another off-target toxicity is the development of B-cell aplasia, a surrogate for CAR T-cell persistence, results in agammaglobulinemia, and requires long-term immunoglobulin replacement [172]. With the use of CD19 directed CART cells, there is a risk of CD19 negative relapse [177]. Trials are underway to study the efficacy of CD22 CART cells as well as the use of dual CARS (CD19 + CD22).

4.2.14 Liposomal drug formulations

The outcomes for pediatric ALL have significantly improved over the past five decades, and the focus is now on minimizing the toxicity and the late effects of chemotherapy. Liposomal doxorubicin has shown remarkably low non-hematological toxicity, although the infection rates may be significant due to severe myelosuppression [178, 179]. In an attempt to decrease the toxicity of therapy, TACL 2012-002 trial is testing the use of liposomal vincristine in children and AYA with relapsed ALL [180]. This study attempts to study the feasibility and safety of liposomal formulation of vincristine sulphate over standard vincristine in first, second or third relapse of B or T ALL.

5. Conclusions and future directions

Treatment of childhood ALL has evolved over the last 50 years with progress made both in the diagnostic and therapeutic arenas. A growing understanding of the biology of the disease has allowed better risk stratification and in some cases alterations to therapy to improve outcomes. Use of pediatric-type protocols in AYA ALL has improved outcomes. Break-through research leading to the development of CAR T-cell therapy, TKIs and monoclonal antibodies have brought a paradigm shift in the management of r/r B ALL. The medical community must now consider the significant cost of these therapies, with questions related to cost-effectiveness and resource allocation ripe for study. Long-term follow-up data for these revolutionary new cancer therapies are required. Outcomes for infant ALL and relapsed T ALL are still dismal and further research is needed to develop newer strategies to combat disease in these group of patients.

Author details

Sneha Tandon and Angela S. Punnett*
Division of Hematology/Oncology, The Hospital for Sick Children, University of Toronto, ON, Canada

*Address all correspondence to: angela.punnett@sickkids.ca

References

[1] Childhood cancer. In: Howlader N, Noone AM, Krapcho M, et al., editors. SEER Cancer Statistics Review, 1975-2010. Bethesda, MD: National Cancer Institute; 2013. Section 28

[2] Childhood cancer by the ICCC. In: Howlader N, Noone AM, Krapcho M, et al., editors. SEER Cancer Statistics Review, 1975-2010. Bethesda, MD: National Cancer Institute; 2013. Section 29

[3] Childhood cancer. In: Howlader N, Noone AM, Krapcho M, et al., editors. SEER Cancer Statistics Review, 1975-2010. Bethesda, MD: National Cancer Institute; 2013. Section 28

[4] Childhood cancer by the ICCC. In: Howlader N, Noone AM, Krapcho M, et al., editors. SEER Cancer Statistics Review, 1975-2010. Bethesda, MD: National Cancer Institute; 2013. Section 29

[5] Bleyer A, O'Leary M, Barr R, Ries LAG, editors. Cancer Epidemiology in Older Adolescents and Young Adults 15-29 Years of Age, Including SEER Incidence and Survival: 1975-2000. National Cancer Institute, NIH Pub.No. 06-5767, Bethesda, MD 2006

[6] Hunger SP, Mullighan GC. Acute lymphoblastic leukemia in children. New England Journal of Medicine. 2015;**373**:1541-1552

[7] Bostrom BC, Sensel MR, Sather HN, et al. Dexamethasone versus prednisone and daily oral versus weekly intravenous mercaptopurine for patients with standard-risk acute lymphoblastic leukemia: A report from the Children's Cancer Group. Blood. 2003;**101**(10):3809-3817

[8] Matloub Y, Bostrom BC, Hunger SP, et al. Escalating intravenous methotrexate improves event-free survival in children with standard-risk acute lymphoblastic leukaemia: A report from the Children's Oncology Group. Blood. 2011;**118**(2):243-251

[9] Seibel NL, Steinherz PG, Sather HN, et al. Early post induction intensification therapy improves survival for children and adolescents with high-risk acute lymphoblastic leukaemia: A report from the Children's Oncology Group. Blood. 2008;**111**(5):2548-2555

[10] Pui CH, Campana D, Pei D, et al. Treating childhood acute lymphoblastic leukemia without cranial irradiation. The New England Journal of Medicine. 2009;**360**(26):2730-2741

[11] Kelly MJ, Trikalinos TA, Dahabreh IJ, Gaianferante M, Parsons SK. Cranial radiation for pediatric acute lymphoblastic leukemia: A systematic review and meta-analysis. American Journal of Hematology. 2014;**89**(10):992-997

[12] Irken G, Oren H, Gulen M, et al. Treatment outcome of adolescents with acute lymphoblastic leukemia. Annals of Hematology. 2002;**81**:641-645

[13] Pui CH, Evans WE. Treatment of acute lymphoblastic leukemia. The New England Journal of Medicine. 2006;**354**:166-178

[14] Stock W, La M, Sanford B, et al. What determines the outcomes for adolescents and young adults with acute lymphoblastic leukemia treated on cooperative group protocols? A comparison of Children's Cancer Group and Cancer and Leukemia Group B studies. Blood. 2008;**112**(5):1646-1654

[15] Boissel N, Auclerc MF, Lhéritier V, et al. Should adolescents with acute lymphoblastic leukemia be treated

as old children or young adults? Comparison of the French FRALLE-93 and LALA-94 trials. Journal of Clinical Oncology. 2003;**21**(5):774-780

[16] van Dongen JJ, Seriu T, Panzer-Grümayer ER, et al. Prognostic value of minimal residual disease in acute lymphoblastic leukaemia in childhood. Lancet. 1998;**352**(9142):1731-1738

[17] Borowitz MJ, Devidas M, Hunger SP, et al. Clinical significance of minimal residual disease in childhood acute lymphoblastic leukemia and its relationship to other prognostic factors: A Children's Oncology Group study. Blood. 2008;**111**(12):5477-5485

[18] Borowitz MJ, Wood BL, Devidas M, et al. Prognostic significance of minimal residual disease in high risk B-ALL: A report from Children's Oncology Group study AALL0232. Blood. 2015;**126**(8):964-971

[19] Möricke A, Zimmermann M, Valsecchi MG, et al. Dexamethasone vs prednisone in induction treatment of paediatric ALL: Results of the randomized trial AIEOP-BFM ALL 2000. Blood. 2016;**127**(17):2101-2112

[20] Vora A, Goulden N, Wade R, et al. Treatment reduction for children and young adults with low-risk acute lymphoblastic leukaemia defined by minimal residual disease (UKALL 2003): A randomized controlled trial. The Lancet Oncology. 2013;**14**(3):199-209

[21] Place AE, Stevenson KE, Vrooman LM, et al. Intravenous pegylated asparaginase versus intramuscular native *Escherichia coli* L-asparaginase in newly diagnosed childhood acute lymphoblastic leukaemia (DFCI 05-001): A randomized, open-label phase 3 trial. The Lancet Oncology. 2015;**16**(16):1677-1690

[22] Pieters R, de Groot-Kruseman H, Van der Velden V, et al. Successful therapy reduction and intensification for childhood acute lymphoblastic leukemia based on minimal residual disease monitoring: Study ALL10 from the Dutch childhood oncology group. Journal of Clinical Oncology. 2016;**34**(22):2591-2601

[23] Wood B, Wu D, Crossley B, et al. Measurable residual disease detection by high-throughput sequencing improves risk stratification for pediatric B-ALL. Blood. 2018;**131**:1350-1359

[24] Vora A, Goulden N, Mitchell C, et al. Augmented post-remission therapy for a minimal residual disease-defined high-risk subgroup of children and young people with clinical standard-risk and intermediate-risk acute lymphoblastic leukaemia (UKALL 2003): A randomized controlled trial. The Lancet Oncology. 2014;**15**(8):809-818

[25] Conter V, Bartram CR, Valsecchi MG, et al. Molecular response to treatment redefines all prognostic factors in children and adolescents with B-cell precursor acute lymphoblastic leukemia: Results in 3184 patients of the AIEOP-BFM ALL 2000 study. Blood. 2010;**115**(16):3206-3214

[26] Tallen G, Ratei R, Mann G, Kaspers G, Niggli F, Karachunsky A, et al. Long-term outcome in children with relapsed acute lymphoblastic leukemia after time-point and site-of-relapse stratification and intensified short-course multidrug chemotherapy: Results of trial ALL-REZ BFM 90. Journal of Clinical Oncology. 2010;**28**:2339-2347

[27] Freyer DR, Devidas M, La M, Carroll WL, Gaynon PS, Hunger SP, et al. Postrelapse survival in childhood acute lymphoblastic leukemia is independent of initial treatment intensity: A report from the

Children's Oncology Group. Blood. 2011;**117**:3010-3015

[28] Arber DA, Orazi A, Hasserjian R, et al. The 2016 revision to the World Health Organization classification of myeloid neoplasms and acute leukemia. Blood. 2016;**127**(20):2391-2405

[29] Pui CH, Relling MV, Downing JR. Acute lymphoblastic leukemia. The New England Journal of Medicine. 2004;**350**:1535-1548

[30] Visscher H, Ross CJ, Rassekh SR, Barhdadi A, et al. Pharmacogenomic prediction of anthracycline-induced cardiotoxicity in children. Journal of Clinical Oncology. 2012;**30**(13):1422-1428

[31] Mullighan CG. Genomic characterization of childhood acute lymphoblastic leukemia. Seminars in Hematology. 2013;**50**(4):314-324

[32] Holmfeldt L, Wei L, Diaz-Flores E, et al. The genomic landscape of hypodiploid acute lymphoblastic leukemia. Nature Genetics. 2013;**45**(3):242-252

[33] Mullighan CG, Miller CB, Radtke I, et al. BCR-ABL1 lymphoblastic leukaemia is characterized by deletion of Ikaros. Nature. 2008;**453**(7191):110-114

[34] Roberts KG, Li Y, Payne-Turner D, et al. Targetable kinase-activating lesions n Ph-like acute lymphoblastic leukaemia. New England Journal of Medicine. 2014;**371**(11):1005-1015

[35] Harvey RC, Mullingham CG, Wang X, et al. Identification of novel cluster groups in pediatric high-risk B-precursor acute lymphoblastic leukemia with gene expression profiling: Correlation with genome-wide DNA copy number alterations, clinical charatcteristics, and outcome. Blood. 2010;**116**(23):4874-4884

[36] Clappier E, Auclerc MF, Rapion J, et al. An intragenic ERG deletion is a marker of an oncogenic subtype of B-cell precursor acute lymphoblastic leukemia with favorable outcome despite frequent IKZF1 deletions. Leukemia. 2014;**28**(1):70-77

[37] Zaliova M, Zimmermannova O, Dorge P, et al. ERG mutation is associated with CD2 and attenuates the negative impact of IKZF1 deletion in childhood acute lymphoblastic leukemia. Leukemia. 2014;**28**(1):182-185

[38] Anderson AK, Ma J, Wang J, et al. The landscape of somatic mutations in infant MLL-rearranged acute lymphoblastic leukemias. Nature Genetics. 2015;**47**(4):330-337

[39] Chillon MC, Gomez-Casares MT, Lopez-Jorge CE, et al. Prognostic significance of FLT-3 mutational status and expression levels in MLL-AF4+ and MLL-germline acute lymphoblastic leukemia. Leukemia. 2012;**26**(11):2360-2366

[40] Stam RW, Schneider P, de Lorenzo P, Valsecchi MG, den Boer ML. Pieters prognostic significance of high-level FLT3 expression in MLL-rearranged infant acute lymphoblastic leukemia. Blood. 2007;**110**(7):2774-2775

[41] Harrison CJ, Moorman AV, Schwab C, et al. An international study of intrachromosomal amplification of chromosome 21 (iAMP21): Cytogenetic characterization and outcome. Leukemia. 2014;**28**(5):1015-1021

[42] Attarbaschi A, Panzer-Grumayer R, Mann G, Moricke A, Konig M, Mecklenbrauker A, et al. Minimal residual disease-based treatment is adequate for relapse-prone childhood acute lymphoblastic leukemia with an intrachromosomal amplification of chromosome 21: The experience of the ALL-BFM 2000 trial. Klinische Pädiatrie. 2014;**226**(6-7):338-343

[43] Gallo Llorente L, Luther H, Schneppenheim R, et al. Identification of novel NOTCH1 mutations: Increasing our knowledge of the NOTCH signaling pathway. Pediatric Blood & Cancer. 2014;**61**(5):788-796

[44] Petit A, Trinquand A, Chevret S, et al. Oncogenetic mutations combined with MRD improve outcome prediction in pediatric T-cell acute lymphoblastic leukemia. Blood. 2018;**131**:289-300

[45] Armstrong SA, Look AT. Molecular genetics of acute lymphoblastic leukaemia. Journal of Clinical Oncology. 2005;**23**(26):6306-6315

[46] Karrman K, Forestier E, Heyman M, et al. Clinical and cytogenetic features of a population-based consecutive series of 285 pediatric T-cell acute lymphoblastic leukemias: Rare T-cell receptor gene rearrangements are associated with poor outcome. Genes, Chromosomes & Cancer. 2009;**48**(9):795-805

[47] Papaemmanuil E, Hosking FJ, Vijayakrishnan J, et al. Loci on 7p12.2, 10q21.2 and 14q11.2 are associated with risk of childhood acute lymphoblastic leukemia. Nature Genetics. 2009;**41**(9):1006-1010

[48] Treviño LR, Yang W, French D, et al. Germline genomic variants associated with childhood acute lymphoblastic leukemia. Nature Genetics. 2009;**41**(9):1001-1005

[49] Migliorini G, Fiege B, Hosking FJ, et al. Variation at 10p12.2 and 10p14 influences risk of childhood B-cell acute lymphoblastic leukemia and phenotype. Blood. 2013;**122**(19):3298-3307

[50] Hungate EA, Vora SR, Gamazon ER, et al. A variant at 9p21.3 functionally implicates CDKN2B in paediatric B-cell precursor acute lymphoblastic leukaemia aetiology. Nature Communications. 2016;7:10635

[51] Sherborne AL, Hosking FJ, Prasad RB, et al. Variation in CDKN2A at 9p21.3 influences childhood acute lymphoblastic leukemia risk. Nature Genetics. 2010;**42**(6):492-494

[52] Xu H, Yang W, Perez-Andreu V, et al. Novel susceptibility variants at 10p12.31-12.2 for childhood acute lymphoblastic leukemia in ethnically diverse populations. Journal of the National Cancer Institute. 2013;**105**(10):733-742

[53] Ellinghaus E, Stanulla M, Richter G, et al. Identification of germline susceptibility loci in ETV6-RUNX1-rearranged childhood acute lymphoblastic leukemia. Leukemia. 2012;**26**(5):902-909

[54] Den Boer ML, van Slegtenhorst M, De Menezes RX, et al. A subtype of childhood acute lymphoblastic leukaemia with poor treatment outcome: A genome-wide classification study. The Lancet Oncology. 2009;**10**(2):125-134

[55] Mullighan CG, Su X, Zhang J, et al. Deletion of IKZF1 and prognosis in acute lymphoblastic leukemia. The New England Journal of Medicine. 2009;**360**(5):470-480

[56] Reshmi SC, Harvey RC, Roberts KG, et al. Targetable kinase gene fusions in high-risk B-ALL: A study from the Children's Oncology Group. Blood. 2017;**129**(25):3352-3361

[57] Kathryn G, Roberts KG, Reshmi SC, Harvey RC, et al. Genomic and outcome analyses of Ph-like ALL in NCI standard-risk patients: A report from the Children's Oncology Group. Blood. 2018;**132**:815-824

[58] Tasian SK, Doral MY, Borowitz MJ, et al. Aberrant STAT5 and PI3K/mTOR pathway signaling occurs in human CRFL2-rearranged B-precursor acute lymphoblastic leukemia. Blood. 2012;**120**(4):833-842

[59] Harvey RC, Mullighan CG, Chen IM, et al. Rearrangement of CRLF2 is associated with mutation of JAK kinases, alteration of IKZF1, Hispanic/Latino ethnicity, and a poor outcome in pediatric B-progenitor acute lymphoblastic leukemia. Blood. 2010;**115**(26):5312-5321

[60] Fang Q, Zhao X, Li Q, et al. IKZF1 alterations and expression of CRLF2 predict prognosis in adult Chinese patients with B-cell precursor acute lymphoblastic leukemia. Leukemia & Lymphoma. 2017;**58**(1):127-137

[61] Dou H, Chen X, Huang Y, et al. Prognostic significance of P2RY8-CRLF2 and CRLF2 overexpression may vary across risk subgroups of childhood B-cell acute lymphoblastic leukemia. Genes, Chromosomes & Cancer. 2017;**56**(2):135-146

[62] Schmäh J, Fedders B, Panzer-Grümayer R, et al. Molecular characterization of acute lymphoblastic leukemia with high CRLF2 gene expression in childhood. Pediatric Blood & Cancer. 2017;**64**:e26539

[63] Schwab CJ, Chilton L, Morrison H, et al. Genes commonly deleted in childhood B-cell precursor acute lymphoblastic leukemia: Association with cytogenetics and clinical features. Haematologica. 2013;**98**(7):1081-1088

[64] Krentz S, Hof J, Mendioroz A, et al. Prognostic value of genetic alterations in children with first bone marrow relapse of childhood B-cell precursor acute lymphoblastic leukemia. Leukemia. 2013;**27**(2):295-304

[65] Feng J, Tang Y. Prognostic significance of IKZF1 alteration status in pediatric B-lineage acute lymphoblastic leukemia: A meta-analysis. Leukemia & Lymphoma. 2013;**54**(4):889-891

[66] Dörge P, Meissner B, Zimmermann M, et al. IKZF1 deletion is an independent predictor of outcome in pediatric acute lymphoblastic leukemia treated according to the ALL-BFM 2000 protocol. Haematologica. 2013;**98**(3):428-432

[67] Olsson L, Castor A, Behrendtz M, et al. Deletions of IKZF1 and SPRED1 are associated with poor prognosis in a population-based series of pediatric B-cell precursor acute lymphoblastic leukemia diagnosed between 1992 and 2011. Leukemia. 2014;**28**(2):302-310

[68] Boer JM, van der Veer A, Rizopoulos D, et al. Prognostic value of rare IKZF1 deletion in childhood B-cell precursor acute lymphoblastic leukemia: An international collaborative study. Leukemia. 2016;**30**(1):32-38

[69] Stanulla M, Dagdan E, Zaliova M, et al. IKZF1plus defines a new minimal residual disease-dependent very-poor prognostic profile in pediatric B-cell precursor acute lymphoblastic leukemia. Journal of Clinical Oncology. 2018;**36**(12):1240-1249

[70] Loh ML, Zhang J, Harvey RC, et al. Tyrosine kinome sequencing of paediatric acute lymphoblastic leukaemia: A report from the Children's Oncology Group TARGET project. Blood. 2013;**121**(3):485-488

[71] Bercovich D, Ganmore I, Scott LM, et al. Muatations of JAK2 in acute lymphoblastic leukaemias associated with down's syndrome. Lancet. 2008;**372**(9648):1484-1492

[72] Roberts KG, Morin RD, Zhang J, et al. Genetic alterations activating kinase and cytokine receptor signaling in high-risk acute lymphoblastic leukemia. Cancer Cell. 2012;**22**(2):153-166

[73] A Phase 2 Study of Ruxolitinib with Chemotherapy in Children with Acute Lymphoblastic Leukemia. ClinicalTrials.gov Identifier: NCT02723994

[74] Russell LJ, Enshaei A, Jones L, et al. IGH translocations are prevalent in teenagers and young adults with acute lymphoblastic leukemia and are associated with a poor outcome. Journal of Clinical Oncology. 2014;**32**(14):1453-1462

[75] Harrison CJ, Haas O, Harbott J, et al. Detection of prognostically relevant genetic abnormalities in childhood B-cell precursor acute lymphoblastic leukemia: Recommendations from the biology and diagnosis Committee of the International Berlin-Frankfurt-Munster study group. British Journal of Haematology. 2010;**151**(2):132-142

[76] Reichard KK, Kang H, Robinson HM, et al. Prognosis of children with acute lymphoblastic leukemia (ALL) and intrachromosomal amplification of chromosome 21 (iAMP21). Blood. 2007;**109**(6):2327-2330

[77] Li Y, Schwab C, Ryan SL, et al. Constitutional and somatic rearrangement of chromosome 21 in acute lymphoblastic leukemia. Nature. 2014;**508**(7494):98-102

[78] Heerema NA, Carroll AJ, Devidas M, et al. Intrachromosomal amplification of chromosome 21 is associated with inferior outcomes in children with acute lymphoblastic leukemia treated in contemporary standard-risk children's oncology group studies: A report from the children's oncology group. Journal of Clinical Oncology. 2013;**31**(27):3397-3402

[79] Moorman AV, Robinson H, Schwab C, et al. Risk-directed treatment intensification significantly reduces the risk of relapse among children and adolescents with acute lymphoblastic leukemia and intrachromosomal amplification of chromosome 21: A comparison of the MRC ALL97/99 and UKALL2003 trials. Journal of Clinical Oncology. 2013;**31**(27):3389-3396

[80] Stock W, La M, Sanford B, et al. What determines the outcome for adolescents and young adults with acute lymphoblastic leukemia treated on cooperative group protocols? A comparison of Children's Cancer Group and Leukemia Group B studies. Blood. 2008;**112**(5):1646-1654

[81] Huguet F, Leguay T, Raffoux E, et al. Pediatric-inspired therapy in adults with Philadelphia chromosome-negative acute lymphoblastic leukemia: The GRALL-2003 study. Journal of Clinical Oncology. 2009;**27**(6):911-918

[82] Advani A, Sanford B, Luger S, et al. Frontline-treatment of acute lymphoblastic leukemia (ALL) In older adolescents and young adults (AYA) using a pediatric regimen is Feaible: Toxicity results of the prospective US intergroup trial C10403(Alliance). Blood. 2013;**122**:903

[83] Testi AM, Valsecchi MG, Conter V, et al. Difference in outcome of adolescents with acute lymphoblastic leukemia (ALL) enrolled in pediatric (AIEOP) and adult (GIMEMA) protocols. [Abstract]. Blood. 2004;**104**:A-1954

[84] de Bont JM, van der Holt B, Dekker AW, et al. Adolescents with acute lymphatic leukaemia achieve significantly better results when treated following Dutch paediatric oncology protocols than with adult protocols. Nederlands Tijdschrift voor Geneeskunde. 2005;**149**(8):400-406

[85] Hallböök H, Gustafsson G, Smedmyr B, et al. Treatment outcome in young adults and children >10 years of age with acute lymphoblastic leukemia in Sweden: A comparison between a pediatric protocol and an adult protocol. Cancer. 2006;**107**(7):1551-1561

[86] Ramanujachar R, Richards S, Hann I, et al. Adolescents with acute lymphoblastic leukaemia: Outcome

on UK national paediatric (ALL97) and adult (UKALLXII/E2993) trials. Pediatric Blood & Cancer. 2007;**48**(3):254-261

[87] Hough R, Rowntree C, Goulden N, et al. Efficacy and toxicity of a paediatric protocol in teenagers and young adults with Philadelphia chromosome negative acute lymphoblastic leukaemia: Results from UKALL 2003. British Journal of Haematology. 2016;**172**(3):439-451

[88] Mullighan CG, Goorha S, Radtke I, et al. Genome-wide analysis of genetic alterations in acute lympoblastic leukemia. Nature. 2007;**446**:758-764

[89] Suryanarayan K, Hunger SP, Kohler S, Carroll AJ, Crist W, Link MP, et al. Consistent involvement of the bcr gener by 9;22 breakpoints in pediatric acute leukemias. Blood. 1991;**77**(2):324-330

[90] Bernt KM, Hunger SP. Current concepts in pediatric Philadelphia chromosome-positive acute lymphoblastic leukemia. Frontiers in Oncology. 2014;**4**:54

[91] Fielding AK, Rowe JM, Buck G, et al. UKALLXII/ECOG2993: Addition of imatinib to a standard treatment regimen enhances long-term outcomes in Philadelphia positive acute lymphoblastic leukemia. Blood. 2014;**123**(6):843-850

[92] Schultz KR, Bowman WP, Aledo A, et al. Improved early event-free survival with imatinib in Philadelphia chromosome-positive acute lymphoblastic leukemia: A children's oncology group study. Journal of Clinical Oncology. 2009;**27**(31):5175-5181

[93] Schultz KR, Carroll A, Heerema NA, et al. Long-term follow-up of imatinib in pediatric Philadelphia chromosome-positive acute lymphoblastic leukemia: Children's oncology group study AALL0031. Leukemia. 2014;**28**(7):1467-1471

[94] Zwaan CM, Rizzari C, Mechinaud F, et al. Dasatinib in children and adolescents with relapsed or refractory leukemia: Results of the CA180-018 phase I dose-escalation study of the Innovative Therapies for Children with Cancer Consortium. Journal of Clinical Oncology. 2013;**31**(19):2460-2468

[95] Kim DY, Joo YD, Lim SN, et al. Nilotinib combined with multiagent chemotherapy for newly diagnosed Philadelphia—Positive acute lymphoblastic leukemia. Blood. 2015;**126**(6):746-756

[96] Ravandi F, Jorgensen JL, Thomas DA, et al. Detection of MRD may predict the outcome of patients with Philadelphia chromosome-positive ALL treated with tyrosine kinase inhibitors plus chemotherapy. Blood. 2013;**122**(7):1214-1221

[97] Giebel S, Czyz A, Ottmann O, et al. Use of tyrosine kinase inhibitors to prevent relapse after allogenic hematopoietic stem cell transplantation for patients with Philadelphia chromosome-positive acute lymphoblastic leukemia. A position statement of the Acute Leukemia Working Party of the European Society for Blood and Marrow Transplantation. Cancer. 2016;**122**(19):2941-2951

[98] ClinicalTrials.gov. International Phase 3 Trial in Philadelphia Chromosome-Positive Acute Lymphoblastic Leukemia. (Ph+ALL) Testing Imatinib in Combination with Two Different Cytotoxic Chemotherapy Backbones. Identifier NCT03007147

[99] Roberts KG, Pei D, Campana D, et al. Outcomes of children with BCR-ABL1-like acute lymphoblastic leukemia treated with risk-directed therapy based on the levels of minimal residual

disease. Journal of Clinical Oncology. 2014;**32**(27):3012-3020

[100] Savino AM, Sarno J, Trentin L, et al. The histone deacetylase inhibitor givinostat (ITF2357) exhibits potent anti-tumor activity against CRF2-rearranged BCP-ALL. Leukemia. 2017;**31**:2365-2375

[101] Kucine N, Marubayashi S, Bhagwat N, et al. Tumor-specific HSP90 inhibition as a therapeutic approach in JAK-mutant acute lymphoblastic leukemias. Blood. 2015;**126**(22):2479-2483

[102] Suryani S, Bracken LS, Harvey RC, et al. Evaluation of the in vitro and in vivo efficacy of the JAK inhibitor AZD1480 against JAK-mutated acute lymphoblastic leukemia. Molecular Cancer Therapeutics. 2015;**14**(2):364-374

[103] Qin H, Cho M, Haso W, et al. Eradication of B-ALL using chimeric antigen receptor-expressing T cells targeting the TSLPR oncoprotein. Blood. 2015;**126**(5):629-639

[104] Wu S-C, Li LS, Kopp N, et al. Activity of the type II JAK2 inhibitor CHZ868 in B-cell acute lymphoblastic leukemia. Cancer Cell. 2015;**28**(1):29-41

[105] Maude SL, Tasian SK, Vincent T, et al. Targeting JAK1/2 and mTOR in murine xenograft models of Ph-like acute lymphoblastic leukemia. Blood. 2012;**120**(17):3510-3518

[106] Tasian SK, Teachey DT, Li Y, et al. Potent efficacy of combined PI3K/mTOR and JAK or ABL inhibition in murine xenograft models of Ph-like acute lymphoblastic leukemia. Blood. 2017;**129**(2):177-187

[107] Richmond J, Robbins A, Evans K, et al. Acute sensitivity of Ph-like acute lymphoblastic leukemia to the SMAC-mimetic birinapant. Cancer Research. 2016;**76**(15):4579-4591

[108] ClinicalTrials.gov. Ruxolitinib or dasatinib with chemotherapy in patients with Philadelphia chromosome (Ph)-like acute lymphoblastic leukemia (ALL). Available from: https://clinicaltrials.gov/ct2/show/NCT02420717.Identifier:NCT02420717

[109] ClinicalTrials.gov. A phase 2 study of ruxolitinib with chemotherapy in children with acute lymphoblastic leukemia. Available from: https://clinicaltrials.gov/ct2/show/NCT02723994. Identifier:NCT02723994

[110] ClinicalTrials.gov. Combination chemotherapy in treating young patients with newly diagnosed high-risk B acute lymphoblastic leukemia and Ph-like TKI sensitive mutations. Available from: http://clinicaltrials.gov/ct2/show/NCT02883049. Identifier:NCT02883049

[111] Harrison CJ, Moorman AV, Broadfield ZJ, et al., Childhood and Adult Leukaemia Working Parties. Three distinct subgroups of hypodiploidy in acute lymphoblastic leukaemia. British Journal of Haematology. 2004;**125**(5):552-559

[112] Nachman JB, Heerema NA, Sather H, et al. Outcome of treatment in children with hypodiploid acute lymphoblastic leukemia. Blood. 2007;**110**(4):1112-1115

[113] McNeer J, Devidas M, Dai Y, Carroll AJ, et al. Hematopoietic stem-cell transplantation does not improve the poor outcome of children with hypodiploid acute lymphoblastic leukemia: A report from Children's Oncology Group. Journal of Clinical Oncology. 2019;**37**:780-789

[114] Safavi S, Paulsson K. Near-haploid and low-hypodiploid acute lymphoblastic leukemia: Two distinct subtypes with consistently poor prognosis. Blood. 2017;**129**(4):420-423

[115] Mullighan CG, Jeha S, Pei D, et al. Outcome of children with hypodiploid ALL treated with risk-directed therapy based on MRD levels. Blood. 2015;**126**(26):2896-2899

[116] Tasian SK, Teachey DT, Rheingold SR. Targeting the PI3K/mTOR pathway in pediatric hematologic malignancies. Frontiers in Oncology. 2014;**4**:108

[117] Mamokin M, Rouce RH, Tashiro H, Brenner MK. A T-cell-directed chimeric antigen receptor for the selective treatment if T-cell malignancies. Blood. 2015;**126**(8):983-992

[118] Hasle H. Pattern of malignant disorders in individuals with Down's syndrome. The Lancet Oncology. 2001;**2**(7):429-436

[119] Whitlock JA. Down syndrome and acute lymphoblastic leukaemia. British Journal of Haematology. 2006;**135**(5):595-602

[120] Zeller B, Gustafsson G, Forestier E, et al. Acute leukaemia in children with Down syndrome: A population-based Nordic study. British Journal of Haematology. 2005;**128**(6):797-804

[121] Buitenkamp TD, Pieters R, Gallimore NE, et al. Outcome in children with Down syndrome and acute lymphoblastic leukaemia: Role of IKZF1 deletions and CRLF2 aberrations. Leukemia. 2012;**26**(10):2204-2211

[122] Hanada I, Terui K, Ikeda F, et al. Gene alterations involving the CRLF2-JAK pathway and recurrent gene deletions in Down syndrome-associated acute lymphoblastic leukemia in Japan. Genes Chromosome Cancer. 2014;**53**(11):902-910

[123] Hertzberg L, Vendramini E, Ganmore I, et al. Down syndrome acute lymphoblastic leukemia, a highly heterogenous disease in which aberrant expression of CRLF2 is associated with mutated JAK2: A report from the International BFM Study Group. Blood. 2010;**115**(5):1006-1017

[124] Gaikwad A, Rye CL, Devidas M, et al. Prevalence and clinical correlates of JAK2 in acute lymphoblastic leukaemia. British Journal of Haematology. 2009;**144**(6):930-932

[125] Heerema NA, Sather HN, Ge J, et al. Cytogenetic studies of infant acute lymphoblastic leukaemia: Poor prognosis of infants with t(4;11)-a report of the Childrens' Cancer Group. Leukemia. 1999;**13**:679-686

[126] Chessells JM, Harrison CJ, Watson SL, Vora AJ, Richards SM. Treatment of infants with lymphoblastic leukaemia: Results of the UK Infant Protocols 1987-1999. British Journal of Haematology. 2002;**117**:306-314

[127] Hilden JM, Dinndorf PA, Meerbaum SO, et al., Children's Oncology Group. Analysis of prognostic factors of acute lymphoblastic leukemia in infants: Report on CCG 1953 from the Children's Oncology Group. Blood. 2006;**108**(2):441-451

[128] Pieters R, Schrappe M, De Lorenzo P, et al. A treatment protocol for infants younger than 1 year with acute lymphoblastic leukemia (Interfant-99): An observational study and a multicentre randomized trial. Lancet. 2007;**370**(9583):240-250

[129] Meyer C, Burmeister T, Groger D, et al. The MLL recombinome of acute leukemias in 2017. Leukemia. 2018;**32**(2):273-284

[130] Taketani T, Taki T, Sugita K, et al. FLT3 mutations in the activation loop of tyrosine kinase domain are frequently found in infant ALL with MLL rearrangements and pediatric

ALL with hyperdiploidy. Blood. 2004;**103**:1085-1088

[131] Armstrong SA, Mabon ME, Silverman LB, et al. FLT3 mutations in childhood acute lymphoblastic leukaemia. Blood. 2003;**103**:3544-3546

[132] Ross ME, Zhou Song G, et al. Classification of paediatric acute lymphoblastic leukaemia by gene expression profiling. Blood. 2003;**102**:2951-2959

[133] Yeoh EJ, Ross ME, Shurtleff SA, et al. Classification, subtype discovery, and prediction of outcome in pediatric acute lymphoblastic leukaemia by gene expression profiling. Cancer Cell. 2002;**1**:13-143

[134] Dreyer ZE, Hilden JM, Jones TL, et al. Intensified chemotherapy without SCT in infant ALL: Results from COG P9407 (Cohort 3). Pediatric Blood & Cancer. 2015 Mar;**62**(3):419-426

[135] Tomizawa D, Koh K, Sato T, et al. Outcome of risk-based therapy for infant acute lymphoblastic leukemia with or without an MLL gene rearrangement, with emphasis on late effects: A final report of two consecutive studies, MLL96 and MLL98, of the Japan Infant Leukemia Study Group. Leukemia. 2007;**21**(11):2258-2263

[136] Stam RW, Schneider P, de Lorenzo P, Valsecchi MG, den Boer ML, Pieters R. Prognostic significance of high-level FLT3 expression in MLL-rearranged infant acute lymphoblastic leukemia. Blood. 2007;**110**(7):2774-2775

[137] ClinicalTrials.gov. A Groupwide Pilot study the Tolerability and Biological Activity of the Addition of Azacytidine (NSC#102816) to Chemotherapy in Infants with acute lymphoblastic leukemia (ALL) and KMT2A(MLL) Gene Rearrangement. Available from: https://clinicaltrials.gov. Identifier:NCT02828358

[138] Patrick K, Wade R, Goulden N, et al. Improved outcomes for children and young people with T-acute lymphoblastic leukaemia: Results of the UKALL2003 Trial. Blood. 2014;**124**(21):3702

[139] Place AE, Stevenson KE, Harris MH, et al. Outcome of childhood T-cell acute lymphoblastic leukemia (T-ALL): Results from DFCI protocol 05-001. ASCO Meeting Abstracts. 2014;**32** (suppl 15):10015

[140] Schrappe M, Valsecchi MG, Bartram CR, et al. Late MRD response determines relapse risk overall and in subsets of childhood T-cell ALL: Results of the AIEOP-BFM-ALL 2000 study. Blood. 2011;**118**(8):2077-2084

[141] Winter SS, Devidas M, Chen S, et al. Capizzi-style methotrexate with pegasparginase (C-MTX) is superior to high-dose methotrexate (HDMTX) in T-lineage acute lymphoblastic leukemia(T-ALL): Results from Children's Oncology Group (COG) AALL0434 [abstract]. Blood. 2015;**126**(23). Abstract 794

[142] Sison EA, Silverman LB. CNS prophylaxis in pediatric acute lymphoblastic leukemia. Hematology. American Society of Hematology. Education Program. 2014;**2014**(1):198-201

[143] Dunsmore KP, Devidas M, Linda SB, et al. Pilot study of nelarabine in combination with intensive chemotherapy in high-risk T-cell acute lymphoblastic leukemia: A report from the Children's Oncology Group. Journal of Clinical Oncology. 2012;**30**(22):2753-2759

[144] Winter SS, Dunsmore KP, Devidas M, et al. Safe integration of nelarabine into intensive chemotherapy in newly diagnosed

T-cell acute lymphoblastic leukemia: Children's Oncology Group Study AALL0434. Pediatric Blood & Cancer. 2015;**62**(7):1176-1183

[145] Raetz EA, Teachey DT. T-cell acute lymphoblastic leukemia. Hematology. 2016;**2016**:580-588

[146] Raetz EA, Borowitz MJ, Devidas M, et al. Reinduction platform for children with first marrow relapse of acute lymphoblastic leukemia. A Children's Oncology Group Study [corrected]. Journal of Clinical Oncology. 2008;**26**(24):3971-3978

[147] Horton T, Lu X, O'Brien M, et al. AALL07P1: Bortezomib with reinduction chemotherapy for first relapse pediatric ALL. A Children's Oncolgy group Study. Pediatric Blood & Cancer. 2014;**61**(S2):S137

[148] Liu Y, Easton J, Shao Y, Maciaszek J, et al. The genomic landscape of pediatric and young adult T-lineage acute lymphoblastic leukemia. Nature Genetics. 2017;**49**(8):1211-1218

[149] Roti G, Stegmaier K. New approaches to target T-ALL. Frontiers in Oncology. 2014;**4**:170

[150] Zhang J, Ding L, Holmfeldt L, et al. The genetic basis of early T-cell precursor acute lymphoblastic leukaemia. Nature. 2012;**481**(7380): 157-163

[151] Gutierrez A, Dahlberg SE, Neuberg DS, et al. Absence of biallelic TCRgamma deletion predicts early treatment failure in pediatric T-cell acute lymphoblastic leukemia. Journal of Clinical Oncology. 2010;**28**(24):3816-3823

[152] Yang YL, Hsiao CC, Chen HY, et al. Absence of biallelic TCRγ deletion predicts induction failure and poorer outcomes in childhood T-cell acute lymphoblastic leukemia. Pediatric Blood & Cancer. 2012;**58**(6):846-851

[153] Durinck K, Goossens S, Peirs S, et al. Novel biological insights in T-cell acute lymphoblastic leukemia. Experimental Hematology. 2015;**8**:625-639

[154] Vincente C, Schwab C, Broux M, et al. Targeted sequencing identifies associations between IL7R-JAK mutations and epigenetic modulators in T-cell acute lymphoblastic leukemia. Haematologica. 2015;**100**(10):1301-1310

[155] Maude SL, Dolai S, Delgado-Martin C, et al. Efficacy of JAK/STAT pathway inhibition in murine xenograft models of early T-cell precursor (ETP) acute lymphoblastic leukemia. Blood. 2015;**125**(11):1759-1767

[156] Patrick K, Wade R, Goulden N, et al. Outcome for children and young people with Early T-cell precursor acute lymphoblastic leukemia treated on a contemporary protocol, UKALL2003. British Journal of Haematology. 2014;**166**(3):421-424

[157] Woods BL, Winter SS, Dunsmore KP, et al. T-lumphoblastic leukemia(T-ALL) shows excellent outcome, lack of significance of the early thymic precursor (ETP) immunophenotype, and validation of the prognostic value of end-induction minimal residual disease (MRD) in Children's Oncology Group (COG) Study AALL0434[abstract]. Blood. 2014;**124**(21).Abstract 1

[158] Kohler G, Milstein C. Continuous cultures of fused cells secreting antibody of predefined specificity. Nature. 1975;**256**:495-497

[159] Nagorsen D, Kufer P, Baeuerle PA, Bargou R. Blinatumomab: A historical perspective. Pharmacology & Therapeutics. 2012;**136**(3):334-342

[160] Topp MS, Gökbuget N, Zugmaier G, et al. Phase II trial of the anti-CD19 bispecific T-cell engager blinatumomab shows hematologic and molecular remissions in patients with relapsed or refractory B-precursor acute lymphoblastic leukemia. Journal of Clinical Oncology. 2014;**32**(36):4134-4140

[161] Gökbuget N, Zugmaier G, Klinger M, et al. Long-term relapse-free survival in a phase 2 study of blinatumomab for the treatment of patients with minimal residual disease in B-Lineage acute lymphoblastic leukemia. Haematologica. 2017;**102**(4):e132-e135

[162] von Stackelberg A, Locatelli F, Zugmaier G, et al. Phase I/phase II study of blinatumomab in pediatric patients with relapsed/refractory acute lymphoblastic leukemia. Journal of Clinical Oncology. 2016;**34**(36):4381-4389

[163] Schlegel P, Lang P, Zugmaier G, et al. Pediatric posttransplant relapsed/refractory B-precursor acute lymphoblastic leukemia shows durable remission by therapy with the T-cell engaging bispecific antibody blinatumomab. Haematologica. 2014;**99**(7):1212-1219

[164] ClinicalTrials.gov. Risk-Stratified Randomized Phase III Testing of Blinatumomab (NSC# 765986) in First Relapse of Childhood B-Lymphoblastic Leukemia (B-ALL). Available from: https://clinicaltrials.gov.Identifier:NCT 02101853

[165] Thomas X. Inotuzumab ozogamicin in the treatment of B-cell acute lymphoblastic leukemia. Expert Opinion on Investigational Drugs. 2012;**21**(16):871-878

[166] Kantarjian H, Ravandi F, Short NJ, et al. Inotuzumab ozogamicin in combination with low-intensity chemotherapy for older patients with Philadelphia chromosome-negative acute lymphoblastic leukemia: A single-arm, phase 2 study. The Lancet Oncology. 2018;**19**(2):240-248

[167] Kantarjian HM, Deangelo DJ, Stelljes M, et al. Inotuzumab ozogamicin versus standard therapy for acute lymphoblastic leukemia. New England Journal of Medicine. 2016;**375**(8):740-753

[168] Calvo C, Brethon B, Hamy CA, Adjaoud D, et al. Inotuzumab ozogamicin compassionate use for the French pediatric patients with relapsed or refractory acute lymphoblastic leukemia. Blood. 2018;**132**:5203

[169] Bhojwani D, Sposto R, Shah NN, Rodriquez V, et al. Inotuzumab ozogamicin in pediatric patients with relapsed/refractory acute lymphoblastic leukemia. Leukemia. 2018

[170] ClinicalTrials.gov. A Phase 2 Study of Inotuzumab Ozogamicin (NSC#772518, IND#TBD) in Children and Young Adults with Relapsed or Refractory CD22+B-Acute Lymphoblastic Leukemia(B-ALL). Identifier: 02981628

[171] Muhammad N, Mao Q, Xia H. CAR T-cells for cancer therapy. Biotechnology & Genetic Engineering Reviews. 2017;**33**(2):190-226

[172] Maude SL, Frey N, Shaw PA, et al. Chimeric antigen receptor T cells for sustained remission in leukemia. The New England Journal of Medicine. 2014;**371**(16):1507-1517

[173] Grupp SA, Laetsch TW, Buechner J. Analysis of a global registration trial of the efficacy and safety of CTL019 in pediatric and young adults with relapsed/refractory acute lymphoblastic leukemia (ALL). Blood. 2016;**128**:221

[174] Maude SL, Pulsipher MA, Boyer MW. Efficacy and safety of CTL019 in the first US phase II multicentre trial in pediatric relapsed/refractory acute leukemia: Results of an interim analysis. Blood. 2016;**128**:2801

[175] Ko RH, Ji L, Barnette P, Bostrom B, Hutchinson R, Raetz E, et al. Outcome of patients treated for relapsed or refractory acute lymphoblastic leukemia: A therapeutic advances in childhood leukemia consortium study. Journal of Clinical Oncology. 2010;**28**:648-654

[176] Maude SL, Laetsch TW, Buechner S, Rives S, et al. Tisagenlecleucel in children and young adults with B-cell lymphoblastic leukemia. New England Journal of Medicine. 2018;**378**:439-448

[177] Grupp SA, Kalos M, Barrett D, et al. Chimeric antigen receptor-modified T cells for acute lymphoid leukemia. The New England Journal of Medicine. 2013;**368**(16):1509-1518

[178] Hunault-Berger M, Leguay T, Thomas X, Legrand O, Huguet F, Bonmati C, et al. A randomized study of pegylated liposomal doxorubicin versus continuous-infusion doxorubicin in elderly patients with acute lymphoblastic leukemia. GRALL-SA1 study. Haematologica. 2011;**96**(2):245-252

[179] Quarello P, Berger M, Rivetti E, Galletto C, Masetti R, et al. FLAG-liposomal doxorubicin (Myocet) regimen for refractory or relapsed acute leukemia pediatric patients. Journal of Pediatric Hematology/Oncology. 2012;**34**(3):208-216

[180] ClinicalTrials.gov. A Pilot Study of Vincristine Sulphate Liposome Injection in Combination with UKALL R3 Induction Chemotherapy for Children, Adolescents, and Young Adults with Relapse of Acute Lymphoblastic Leukemia. Identifier: NCT02879643

Chapter 4

miRNAs in Acute Lymphoblastic Leukemia: Diagnosis, Prognosis and Target Therapeutic

Yazmín Gómez-Gómez, Jorge Organista-Nava, Berenice Illades-Aguiar and Marco Antonio Leyva-Vázquez

Abstract

Acute lymphoblastic leukemia (ALL) is more frequent in children than in adults. The ALL is a hematological neoplasia, which is characterized by the hyperproliferation of lymphoid precursors in bone marrow. MicroRNAs (miRNAs) are a class of noncoding RNAs that regulate mRNA expression at posttranscriptional level. miRNAs regulate different biological processes such as development, proliferation, apoptosis, hematopoiesis, drug resistance, and tumorigenesis. It has also been observed that the expression of miRNAs can be used to the classification of the different subtypes of ALL. Likewise, miRNAs can also be used to determine the prognostic value and may represent potential therapeutic target molecules in the treatment of ALL.

Keywords: miRNAs, acute lymphoblastic leukemia, diagnosis, prognosis, therapy, biomarkers

1. Introduction

The hematopoiesis is primarily regulated at the transcriptional level by transcription factors that act as master regulators of genes expression. However, the transcriptional process alone does not appear to control all aspects of cellular functioning (cell fate, lineage, etc.), suggesting the participation of other mechanisms. The miRNAs constitute another critical way of hematopoietic regulation. The B- and T-lymphocytes develop from progenitor cells that occur in different organs; B-cell lymphopoiesis is completed in the bone marrow, whereas T-cell lymphopoiesis occurs in the thymus. However, their development and activation are controlled by signaling pathways, which are also regulated by the microRNAs (miRNAs) [1]. miRNA expression profile during the normal and malignant hematopoiesis suggests that miRNAs are regulators of hematopoiesis implicated in regulating and maintenance of the "stemness" of the early progenitors, various stages of cell differentiation, and malignance [2].

Nowadays, there is evidence that miRNAs do not just regulate hematopoietic differentiation and proliferation but also their activity. Deregulation of the expression of miRNAs has been observed in leukemias, and mechanistic studies reveal a role for miRNAs in the pathogenesis of this disorder [3].

IntechOpen

Leukemia is a clonal disorder in which the normal hematopoiesis is replaced by a malignant clonal expansion of immature hematopoietic cells (blasts) in the bone marrow or peripheral blood [4]. The first approach between miRNAs and leukemia was carried out by Calin et al. [5]. The author showed that the 13q14 deletion in B-cell chronic lymphocytic leukemias (B-CLLs) causes the loss of the precursor gene of miR-16-1 and miR-15a; therefore, the loss of these miRNAs is observed in approximately 70% of the CLLs [5]. Interestingly, it has been reported that at fragile sites, minimal regions of amplification (minimal amplicons), or common break-point regions fragile sites, minimal regions of loss of heterozygosity, and genomic regions related with cancer code for approximately 50% of the miRNAs, hence the aberrant expression of different miRNAs in cancer [6].

The participation of miRNAs in different biological and cellular processes under pathological and normal conditions makes them good candidates in the investigation of functional markers for differential diagnosis, prognosis, and development of new therapeutic regimens, through the investigation of their molecular targets. In this chapter, the role of miRNAs expression profiles in ALL that could be used for classification of the disease establishing specific diagnoses and prognostic values is summarized. Likewise, the relation between the miRNA dysregulation and ALL may be a potential therapeutic target.

2. MiRNA biogenesis

The miRNA genes are transcribed by RNA polymerase II (Pol II) in the nucleus, and the primary miRNAs transcripts (pri-miRNAs) contain cap structures as well as poly(A) tails [7, 8]. The pri-miRNA transcript is processed by the microprocessor complex (Drosha/DGCR8), which crops the pri-miRNAs, producing a pre-miRNA

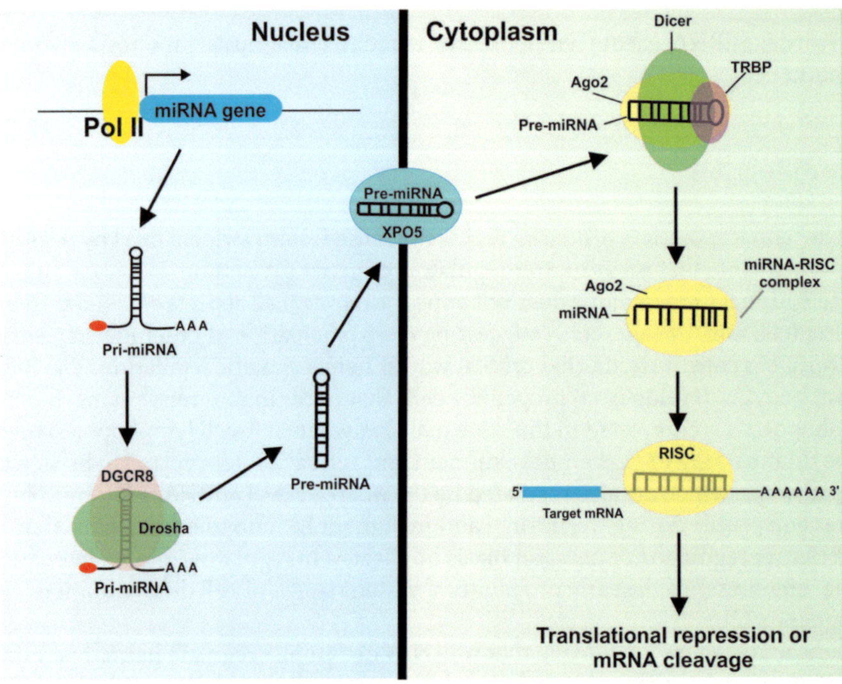

Figure 1.
miRNA biogenesis.

(transcript of about 70 kb) [9–11]. The exportin 5 (XPO5) mediates the export of the pre-miRNAs from the nucleus to the cytoplasm [12–14]. In the cytosol, the pre-miRNA is recognized by Dicer enzyme (RNAse type III), producing a mature **miRNA duplexes** (miRNA:miRNA*) about 22 nucleotides [10]. The miRNA duplex binds to the RNA-induced silencing complex (RISC) [which is composed by of the transactivation-responsive RNA-binding protein (TRBP) and Argonaute2 (Ago2)] [8, 15]. The mature strand is retained by the Ago2 protein in the RISC complex, who directs the mature mRNA to its mRNA target for posttranscriptional gene silencing, while the complementary strand is degraded [16, 17] (**Figure 1**).

3. Functions of the miRNAs in lymphopoiesis

Lymphopoiesis is a process by which the hematopoietic stem cells (HSCs) differentiate into lymphoid progenitors and finally into B- or T-lymphocytes [18]. In the process of differentiation, the miRNAs play an important role. miR-29a and miR-196b are highly expressed by HSCs, and their downregulation is associated with differentiation into lymphoid progenitors [19, 20]. It has been reported that miR-17, miR-24, miR-155, miR-128, and miR-181 act to prevent the differentiation of early-stage progenitors [21].

miRNA-150 is expressed in both mature B- and T-cells. The lymphoid progenitors express the miRNA-150 to give rise to the mature B-cells and assist in the transition from progenitor B-cell (pro-B) to the precursor B-cell (pre-B) stage [18]. And premature expression of miRNA-150 results in blocked transition from the pro-B-cell stage to the pre-B-cell stage [22, 23].

B-cell differentiation is regulated by the miR-155, and it has been observed that miR-155 levels are upregulated rapidly in both activated mature T- and B-cells [24]. Also, miRNA-155 regulates the differentiation of T-cells into Th type 1 cells [24, 25].

miR-181 is specifically expressed in hematopoietic cell, and its expression is dynamically regulated during early hematopoiesis and lineage commitment. miR-181 expression is high in the early B-cell differentiation stage and progressively decreases subsequently, and its ectopic expression in hematopoietic stem/progenitor cells led to an increased fraction of B-lineage cells in both tissue culture differentiation assays and adult mice [26]. Additionally, miR-181 also plays an important role in T-cell development [27].

The miRNA-15 family is an element required to promote the switch from pre-B-cell proliferation to a more differentiated stage. [28]. So, pre-B-cells lacking miRNA-15 family functions exhibit prolonged proliferation because of aberrant expression of the target genes cyclin E1 and D3, and they additionally fail to trigger the transcriptional reprogramming normal to their differentiation, resulting in a developmental block at the pre-B-cell stage [28].

Six miRNAs, miR-17, miR-18a, miR-19a, miR-20a, miR-19b-1, and miR-92a-1 are part of the miR-17-92 cluster; these small molecules are important for mature B-cell development. Absence of the cluster leads to the development of disorders in the maturation from pro-B to pre-B stage [29]. Ventura et al. using miR-17-92-deficient mice found that B-cell development is inhibited at the pro-B to pre-B stage differentiation [30]. The above shows that if the miR-17-92 family miRNAs control the pro- to pre-B transition during B-cell development [31]. Likewise, it has been showed that in helper T cells, the miR-17–92a cluster is critical for the differentiation from Th1 cells [32].

miR-29b is increased in Th1 cells, and the levels from this miRNA decrease significantly upon T cell activation. So, the miR-29 expression can serve as a regulator of Th1 differentiation [33]. Expression of miR-21 promotes Th2 differentiation in nonpolarized T cells [34]. miR-126 is another miRNA that also regulates the differentiation of the Th2 cells [35].

4. miRNA expression and its role in the differential diagnosis of acute lymphoblastic leukemia subtypes

Acute lymphoblastic leukemia (ALL) is characterized by clonal proliferation of early B- and T-lymphocyte progenitors that result in the accumulation of lymphoblasts in the bone marrow and various extramedullary sites. ALL is also the hematology neoplasia most commonly observed in the pediatric population, while it is relatively **less common than AML** in adults [36]. Around 75% of childhood ALL cases contain at least one alteration chromosomic, have lymphoid maturation arrest in distinct stages, and involve B- or T-lineages to leaving different immunophenotypes with different miRNA signatures [37].

microRNAs participate in different physiological and cellular processes, such as development and tissue differentiation, cell identity, cell cycle progression, and programmed cell death [38]. Nowadays, it is known that the distinct stages of lymphopoiesis and the direction of lymphoid precursor maturation are influenced by miRNA expression differentially. However, an aberrant expression of miRNAs is related with malignant lymphopoiesis, characteristic that can be utilized as signature to diagnosis and classification diagnosis of acute lymphoblastic leukemia [18]. Interestingly, miRNA groups that can clearly differentiate ALL of its normal counterpart, B-ALL versus T-ALL and ALL subtypes with specific genetic abnormalities have been reported. De Oliveira and collaborators reported miRNA-128a and miRNA-181b overexpressed and miRNA-100, miRNA-196b, and let-7e with lower level when compared the miRNAs expression in normal pediatric bone morrow (BM) samples and BM samples of pediatric ALL. The authors point out miR-196b as a miRNA highly expressed in T-ALL, while miR-100 was related with the presence of t(12;21) [39].

A study in Brazilian children with T- or B-cell acute lymphoblastic leukemia (T-ALL or B-ALL) evaluated a bone marrow miRNAs profile that may be used for distinguishing childhood lymphoblastic leukemia subtypes [40]. The authors mention that miR-708-5p, miR-497-5p, miR-151a-5p, miR-151b, miR-371b-5p, miR-455-5p, miR-195-5p, miR-1266-5p, miR-574-5p, miR-425-5p downregulated and miR-450b-5p, miR-450a-5p, miR-542-5p, miR-424-5p, miR-629-5p, miR-29c-5p upregulated in childhood T-ALL may be used for distinguishing childhood T- and B-ALL subtypes. However, a machine learning analysis showed that miR-29c-5p, which is involved in calcium signaling, is critical for B-cell lymphocyte fate. So, it is the best discriminator between childhood T- and B-ALL [40].

In a series of adult ALL cases, the expression profile of 470 miRNAs was measured by microarray analysis; 3 miRNAs (miR-148, miR-151, and miR-424) were identified as discriminative of T-lineage versus B-lineage ALL; and miR-151 dramatically downmodulated an miR-148a and miR-424 with higher expression in patients with T-ALL [41]. Furthermore, in the B-lineage ALL cases with special molecular lesions, those with BCR/ABL, E2A/PBX1, MLL/AF4 rearrangements and cases lacking known genetic abnormalities can be differentiated by a set of six miRNA, which was highlighted by one-way analysis of variance [41]. These miRNAs were preferentially expressed in each chromosomic rearrangement; miR-425-5p, miR-191, and miR-128 were expressed in the E2A/PBX1-positive case, miR-629 was highly expressed in cases harboring MLL/AF4 rearrangement, while high levels of miR-146b and miR-126 were observed in the BCR/ABL-positive cases [41]. Other study in pediatric ALL showed

ALL subtype	Upregulated expression	Downregulated expression	References
Children			
T-ALL	miR-450b-5p, miR-450a-5p, miR-542-5p, miR-424-5p, miR-629-5p, miR-29c-5p	miR-708-5p, miR-497-5p, miR-151a-5p, miR-151b, miR-371b-5p, miR-455-5p, miR-195-5p, miR-1266-5p, miR-574-5p, miR-425-5p	[39]
MLL-rearranged, T-ALL	miR-196b		[41]
TEL-AML1 BCR-ABL, E2A-PBX1, hyperdiploid, and B-other	miRNA-708		
Adults			
T-ALL	miR-148a, miR-424	miR-151	[40]
E2A/PBX1-positive B-ALL	miR-425-5p, miR-191, miR-128		
MLL/AF4-positive B-ALL	miR-629		
BCR/ABL-positive B-ALL	miR-146b, miR-126		

Table 1.
Expression of miRNAs in children and adults to differentiate acute lymphoblastic leukemia subtypes.

in seven major subtypes of pediatric ALL, which included: T-cell, MLL-rearranged, TEL-AML1-positive, E2A-PBX1-positive, hyperdiploid ALL, BCR-ABL-positive, and B-other ALLs, the differential miRNA expression. miRNA-708 was highly expressed in TEL-AML1, BCR-ABL, E2A-PBX1, hyperdiploid, and B-other cases than in the MLL-rearranged and T-ALL cases. On the other hand, the expression of miR-196b was higher in MLL-rearranged and T-ALL cases as compared with the expression level in the precursor B-ALL cases [42]. This information suggests that upregulated expression of miR-424 and downregulated expression of miR-151 might be good diagnostic markers to differentiate T-ALL regardless of age (**Table 1**).

Malik and collaborators propose a novel miR-2909-KLF4 molecular axis to differentiate the pathogeneses of pediatric B- and T-cell ALLs that may represent a new diagnostic marker, through alterations in miRNA expression patterns and their respective targets. The authors demonstrate the ability of miR-2909 to repress KLF4 expression in pediatric B-ALL, but not T-ALL [43]. Another interesting work shows that miR-19b, miR-20a, miR-26a, miR-92, and miR-223 have cooperative effects on tumor suppressor genes implicated in the pathogenesis of T-ALL, including *IKAROS*, *PTEN*, *BIM*, *PHF6*, *NF1*, and *FBXW7*. Interestingly, these miRNAs are capable of promoting T-ALL development in a mouse model [44].

5. MicroRNAs as prognostic markers in ALL

MiRNAs are suggested as promising biomarkers not only in the diagnosis but also in the prognosis of ALL patients. Since they have been promising in identifying subgroups of patients with different clinical outcomes [45]. It has been observed that ectopic expression of miRNAs leads to the development of leukemia, such is the case of miR-125b, which has been reported in mice transplanted with fetal liver cells ectopically expressing miR-125b that showed an increase in white blood cell count, in particular in neutrophils and monocytes, associated with a macrocytic anemia. These mice developed B-cell acute lymphoblastic leukemia, T-cell acute lymphoblastic leukemia, or a myeloproliferative neoplasm, suggesting an important role for miR-125b in early hematopoiesis [46].

Patients group with high miR-21 expression was significantly associated with those aged <2 and > 10 years, lower platelets count, more incidence of central nervous system (CNS) infiltration, and poorer treatment outcome also; patients with high miR-21 showed a significantly poorer disease-free survival (DFS) and overall survival (OS) compared with those with low miR-21 expression group [47]. Also, miR-92a expression is significantly higher in ALL compared with peripheral blood mononuclear cells (PBMNCs) from healthy volunteers. Likewise, the expression levels of miR-99a, miR-100, and miR-128b correlated high-risk prognostic factors, including white blood cell (WBC) count, ALL subclassification (T-cell and B-cell ALL), the MLL-rearranged gene, and the BCR-ABL fusion gene, suggesting possible relation of miR-99a, miR-100, and miR-218b with prognosis [48, 49]. It has also been reported that mir-125b-2 is highly expressed in childhood ETV6/RUNX1 (TEL/AML1) leukemias and confers survival advantage to growth inhibitory signals independent of p53 [50].

More specifically, miR-9, miR-24, and miR-92a expression was significantly increased in a subset of ALL cells, and ALL patients with overexpressed miR-24 and miR-92a had poor prognoses [51–53]. Wang et al. (2010) observed that miR-146a, miR-181a/c, and miR-221 were significantly associated with overall survival of the ALL patients. Expression level of miR-146a and miR-181a/c was associated with a poor outcome (i.e., poor prognosis/short-term survival), whereas that of miR-221 was associated with a good outcome (i.e., good prognosis/long-term survival) [54], while that of miR-423-5p is associated with a poorer survival in patients with ALL [55]. Otherwise, the reduced expression of miR-155, miR-181b, miR-182, miR-143, miR-210, and miR-335 is associated with poor outcome of pediatric ALL [56–60]. Also, the expression of miRNAs miR-18a, miR-532, miR-218, miR-625, miR-193a, miR-638, miR-550, and miR-633 is associated with early relapse in childhood ALL, suggesting possible relation of these miRNAs with prognosis [61].

The high miR-16 expression is associated with hyperleukocytosis and poor cytogenetic groups. In B-cell ALL patients, the DFS was significantly shorter in patients with high miR-16 levels. While in T-cell ALL patients, for both DFS and overall survival, a significant trend was found with a survival shortening from the lowest to the highest miR-16 levels [62, 63]. Likewise, it was reported that the expression of miR-16 was upregulated in cases of T lymphoblastic lymphoma/leukemia (T-LBL/ALL), and the high expression group of miR-16 was significantly correlated with longer over survival [64].

For instance, Gimenes-Teixeira et al. reported that T-ALL patients with high miR-221 expression had significantly lower 5-year overall survival (OS) rates compared with those with low miR-221 expression [65]. Oliveira et al. observed that lower levels of miR-29a were significantly associated with higher blast counts in the bone marrow and with increased disease-free survival in T-ALL patients [66].

6. miRNAs in response to commonly used chemotherapy agents in pediatric acute lymphoblastic leukemia

Despite the great effort of current treatment strategies, drug resistance still remains a major cause of chemotherapy failure and relapse in pediatric patients.

miRNAs have not only become tools for classifying subtypes of ALL and in support of the prognosis of this disease, but also studies have reported the classification of patients sensitive or resistant to drugs based on the expression of miRNAs.

Glucocorticoids (GCs) regulate proliferation, differentiation, metabolism, and cell survival in many tissues. In lymphocytes, they affect cell cycle progression, influence immunoglobulin and lymphokine production, and induce apoptosis in immature lymphoblasts [67]. Actually, these drugs are used clinically in the treatment of childhood acute lymphoblastic leukemia (ALL) and other lymphoid malignancies. In the group of glucocorticoids that is administered to patients with ALL is the prednisone; unfortunately, a proportion of patients are insensitive to this drug. A study in 49 ALL patients showed that miR-18a, miR-532, miR-218, miR-625, miR-193a, miR-638, miR-550, and miR-633 could distinguish prednisone-sensitive patients from prednisone-insensitive patients [68]. In contrast, other authors in a group of 81 children with newly diagnosed ALL, no discriminative microRNAs were found for prednisolone response [69].

It is well known that the presence of translocations in ALL is a frequent and prognostic influence event. In leukemia, MLL rearrangements are a common genetic alteration; MLL-AF4 acute lymphocytic leukemia (ALL), resulting from a balanced translocation between *MLL* and *AF4,* occurs in approximately 50% of ALL cases in infants, 2% in children, and 5–6% in adults. The poor prognosis of MLL-AF4 ALL to glucocorticoid-induced apoptosis is associated with its resistance to this drug [70]. miR-128b and miR-221 are commonly downregulated in MLL-rearranged ALL compared with other types of ALL; also these miRNAs downregulate mRNAs encoding CDKN1B, MLL, AF4, and both MLL-AF4 and AF4-MLL fusion genes that are thought to contribute to leukemia development [71]. Interestingly, the restoration of miRNA-128b downregulates target genes including *MLL*, *AF4*, and both *MLL-AF4* and *AF4-MLL* fusion oncogenes, and the restoration of miRNA-221 downregulates CDKN1B cooperatively. Thus, the sensitivity of MLL-AF4 ALL cells to GCs is strengthened [71]. Study developed by Kotani et al. supports the idea that restoration of miRNA-128b improves the sensitivity of MLL-AF4 ALL cells to GCs. This author mentioned that one novel mutation of miRNA-128b significantly reduced its processing, and the resultant downregulation of mature miRNA-128b gave rise to GCs resistance due to the failure to downregulate the fusion oncogenes [72]. This suggests that miRNA-128b and miRNA-221 could be GC (dexamethasone) sensitizers potential.

Other microRNAs related with drug resistance in pediatric acute lymphoblastic leukemia are miR-454, which present a low expression in L-asparaginase-resistant cases, whereas miR-125b, miR-99a, and miR-100 show an upregulation of their expression in patients resistant to vincristine and daunorubicin [69].

7. miRNAs as therapeutic targets in acute lymphoblastic leukemia

Nowadays, advances in our understanding of the molecular carcinogenesis of the human cancers and the extensive research on generate and implement new combined and targeted therapies, and have allowed to know specific molecular therapeutic targets. However, there is still a continuous need for development of new therapeutic tools for applicability.

RNA molecules actually are the therapeutic targets promising in the molecular oncology. The ability of miRNAs to regulate important cellular processes, by concurrently regulating multiple targets, their inherent role in carcinogenesis as oncogenes or tumor suppressor genes, and the aberrant dysregulation of their expression levels in cancer, can represent a viable therapeutic strategy and a powerful intervention tool in **leukemia** [73]. For example, in leukemia cells isolated from individuals with BCR/ABL, TKI-resistant Philadelphia-chromosome-positive acute lymphoblastic leukemia (Ph + ALL) was observed an increase in levels of DNMT3A in association with downregulation of miR-217; these observations are clinically relevant; and inhibition of DNMT3A by forced expression of miRNA-217 may benefit in preventing drug resistance to TKI treatment in Philadelphia-chromosome-positive ALL patients [74]. Another therapeutic strategy for BCR-ABL-positive ALL is miRNA-203, which has as direct target to BCR-ABL1 and ABL1, proteins with activity tyrosine kinase. This miRNA is silenced by genetic and epigenetic mechanisms in hematopoietic malignancies expressing either ABL1 or BCR-ABL1. However, the restoration of the miRNA-203 expression reduces ABL1 and BCR-ABL1 levels and inhibits cell proliferation [75]. miRNA-143 was identified as a regulator of MLL-AF4 expression and is epigenetically repressed by promoter hypermethylation in MLL-AF4-positive primary blasts and cell lines;upregulation of miRNA-143 expression by demethylation has therapeutic promise for MLL-AF4 B-cell ALL [76].

It is also important to consider that some miRNAs can behave as oncogenes in one cancer type and as tumor suppressive genes in others. It has been reported that miR-221 maintains a high expression in hepatic cancer and exerts an oncogenic function by targeting tumor suppressor PTEN, but this miRNA acts as a tumor suppressor in erythroblastic leukemia by inhibiting the KIT oncogene expression [77, 78]. Thus, identification of specific biological functions, type of cancer, and targets of miRNAs is a basic aspect when considering miRNA therapeutics.

8. Summary and future directions

Various studies have demonstrated that the oncomiRs or tumor suppressor miRNAs expression may significantly have potential how diagnostic and/or prognostic biomarkers, as well as monitoring the disease progression and in the response to treatment, and it may be a therapeutic target for treatment in ALL. Also, miRNAs expression levels may play an important role in the genesis and evolution of the ALL. Nevertheless, the biological effects and relevant target genes of many miRNAs that are deregulated and/or prognostically relevant in ALL need to be identified and characterized. Therefore, novel anti-ALL agents are needed to overcome chemotherapy resistance and reduce cytotoxicity. The mimics- and/or anti-miRNAs may be a good alternative. However, more experiments are required to evaluate the feasibility and safety of mimics- and/or anti-miRNAs in the clinical treatment.

Acknowledgements

This work was supported by the Universidad Autónoma de Guerrero. Yazmín Gómez-Gómez (CVU: 236728) and Jorge Organista-Nava (CVU: 236745) were recipient of postdoctoral fellowships from CONACYT.

Conflict of interest

The authors declare that there are no conflicts of interest.

Author details

Yazmín Gómez-Gómez†, Jorge Organista-Nava*†, Berenice Illades-Aguiar and Marco Antonio Leyva-Vázquez*
Molecular Biomedicine Laboratory, School of Chemical-Biological Sciences, Autonomous University of Guerrero, Chilpancingo, Guerrero, Mexico

*Address all correspondence to: leyvamarco13@gmail.com and joorna@gmail.com

† These authors contributed equally to this work

References

[1] Johanson TM, Skinner JPJ, Kumar A, Zhan Y, Lew AM, Chong MMW. The role of microRNAs in lymphopoiesis. International Journal of Hematology. 2014;**100**(3):246-253. DOI: 10.1007/s12185-014-1606-y

[2] Ultimo S, Martelli AM, Zauli G, Vitale M, Calin GA, Neri LM. Roles and clinical implications of MicroRNAs in acute lymphoblastic leukemia. Journal of Cellular Physiology. 2018;**233**(8):5642-5654. DOI: 10.1002/jcp.26290

[3] Garzon R, Croce CM. MicroRNAs in normal and malignant hematopoiesis. Current Opinion in Hematology. 2008;**15**(4):352-358. DOI: 10.1097/MOH.0b013e328303e15d

[4] Zhao H, Wang D, Du W, Gu D, Yang R. MicroRNA and leukemia: Tiny molecule, great function. Critical Reviews in Oncology/Hematology. 2010;**74**(3):149-155. DOI: 10.1016/j.critrevonc.2009.05.001

[5] Calin GA, Dumitru CD, Shimizu M, Bichi R, Zupo S, Noch E, et al. Frequent deletions and down-regulation of micro- RNA genes miR15 and miR16 at 13q14 in chronic lymphocytic leukemia. Proceedings of the National Academy of Sciences of the United States of America. 2002;**99**(24):15524-15529. DOI: 10.1073/pnas.242606799

[6] Calin GA, Sevignani C, Dumitru CD, Hyslop T, Noch E, Yendamuri S, et al. Human microRNA genes are frequently located at fragile sites and genomic regions involved in cancers. Proceedings of the National Academy of Sciences of the United States of America. 2004;**101**(9):2999-3004. DOI: 10.1073/pnas.0307323101

[7] Lee Y, Kim M, Han J, Yeom K-H, Lee S, Baek SH, et al. MicroRNA genes are transcribed by RNA polymerase II. The EMBO Journal. 2004;**23**(20):4051-4060. DOI: 10.1038/sj.emboj.7600385

[8] Lin S, Gregory RI. MicroRNA biogenesis pathways in cancer. Nature Reviews Cancer. 2015;**15**(6):321-333. DOI: 10.1038/nrc3932

[9] Han J, Lee Y, Yeom K-H, Kim Y-K, Jin H, Kim VN. The Drosha-DGCR8 complex in primary microRNA processing. Genes & Development. 2004;**18**(24):3016-3027. DOI: 10.1101/gad.1262504

[10] Acunzo M, Romano G, Wernicke D, Croce CM. MicroRNA and cancer—A brief overview. Advances in Biological Regulation. 2015;**57**:1-9. DOI: 10.1016/j.jbior.2014.09.013

[11] Wu Q, Song R, Ortogero N, Zheng H, Evanoff R, Small CL, et al. The RNase III enzyme DROSHA is essential for microRNA production and spermatogenesis. The Journal of Biological Chemistry. 2012;**287**(30):25173-25190. DOI: 10.1074/jbc.M112.362053

[12] Kim VN. MicroRNA precursors in motion: Exportin-5 mediates their nuclear export. Trends in Cell Biology. 2004;**14**(4):156-159. DOI: 10.1016/j.tcb.2004.02.006

[13] Yi R, Qin Y, Macara IG, Cullen BR. Exportin-5 mediates the nuclear export of pre-microRNAs and short hairpin RNAs. Genes & Development. 2003;**17**(24):3011-3016. DOI: 10.1101/gad.1158803

[14] Bohnsack MT, Czaplinski K, Gorlich D. Exportin 5 is a RanGTP-dependent dsRNA-binding protein that mediates nuclear export of pre-miRNAs. RNA. 2004;**10**(2):185-191. DOI: 10.1261/rna.5167604

[15] Chendrimada TP, Gregory RI, Kumaraswamy E, Norman J, Cooch N, Nishikura K, et al. TRBP recruits the Dicer complex to Ago2 for microRNA processing and gene silencing. Nature. 2005;**436**(7051):740-744. DOI: 10.1038/nature03868

[16] Bartel DP. MicroRNAs: Genomics, biogenesis, mechanism, and function. Cell. 2004;**116**(2):281-297. DOI: 10.1016/S0092-8674(04)00045-5

[17] Diederichs S, Haber DA. Dual role for argonautes in microRNA processing and posttranscriptional regulation of microRNA expression. Cell. 2007;**131**(6):1097-1108. DOI: 10.1016/j.cell.2007.10.032

[18] Luan C, Yang Z, Chen B. The functional role of microRNA in acute lymphoblastic leukemia: Relevance for diagnosis, differential diagnosis, prognosis, and therapy. OncoTargets and Therapy. 2015;**8**:2903-2914. DOI: 10.2147/OTT.S92470

[19] Han Y-C, Park CY, Bhagat G, Zhang J, Wang Y, Fan J-B, et al. microRNA-29a induces aberrant self-renewal capacity in hematopoietic progenitors, biased myeloid development, and acute myeloid leukemia. Journal of Experimental Medicine. 2010;**207**(3):475-489. DOI: 10.1084/jem.20090831

[20] Popovic R, Riesbeck LE, Velu CS, Chaubey A, Zhang J, Achille NJ, et al. Regulation of mir-196b by MLL and its overexpression by MLL fusions contributes to immortalization. Blood. 2009;**113**(14):3314-3322. DOI: 10.1182/blood-2008-04-154310

[21] Manterola L, Fernandez-Mercado M, Larrea E, Goicoechea I, Arestin M, Armesto M, et al. MicroRNAs as B-cell lymphoma biomarkers. Blood and Lymphatic Cancer: Targets and Therapy. 2015;**5**:25-34. DOI: 10.2147/BLCTT.S60481

[22] Zhou B, Wang S, Mayr C, Bartel DP, Lodish HF. miR-150, a microRNA expressed in mature B and T cells, blocks early B cell development when expressed prematurely. Proceedings of the National Academy of Sciences of the United States of America. 2007;**104**(17):7080-7085. DOI: 10.1073/pnas.0702409104

[23] He Y, Jiang X, Chen J. The role of miR-150 in normal and malignant hematopoiesis. Oncogene. 2014;**33**(30):3887-3893. DOI: 10.1038/onc.2013.346

[24] Seddiki N, Brezar V, Ruffin N, Lévy Y, Swaminathan S. Role of mi R-155 in the regulation of lymphocyte immune function and disease. Immunology. 2014;**142**(1):32-38. DOI: 10.1111/imm.12227

[25] Banerjee A, Schambach F, DeJong CS, Hammond SM, Reiner SL. Micro RNA-155 inhibits IFN-γ signaling in CD4+ T cells. European Journal of Immunology. 2010;**40**(1):225-231. DOI: 10.1002/eji.200939381

[26] Chen C-Z, Li L, Lodish HF, Bartel DP. MicroRNAs modulate hematopoietic lineage differentiation. Science. 2004;**303**(5654):83-86. DOI: 10.1126/science.1091903

[27] Verduci L, Azzalin G, Gioiosa S, Carissimi C, Laudadio I, Fulci V, et al. microRNA-181a enhances cell proliferation in acute lymphoblastic leukemia by targeting EGR1. Leukemia Research. 2015;**39**(4):479-485. DOI: 10.1016/j.leukres.2015.01.010

[28] Lindner SE, Lohmüller M, Kotkamp B, Schuler F, Knust Z, Villunger A, et al. The miR-15 family reinforces the transition from proliferation to differentiation in pre-B cells. EMBO Reports. 2017;**18**(9):1604-1617. DOI: 10.15252/embr.201643735

[29] Violaine H, Ramiro G. Micrornas: Emerging key regulators of hematopoiesis. American Journal of Hematology. 2010;**85**(12):935-942. DOI: 10.1002/ajh.21863

[30] Ventura A, Young AG, Winslow MM, Lintault L, Meissner A, Erkeland SJ, et al. Targeted deletion reveals essential and overlapping functions of the miR-17~92 family of miRNA clusters. Cell. 2008;**132**(5):875-886. DOI: 10.1016/j.cell.2008.02.019

[31] Lai M, Gonzalez-Martin A, Cooper AB, Oda H, Jin HY, Shepherd J, et al. Regulation of B-cell development and tolerance by different members of the miR-17~92 family microRNAs. Nature Communications. 2016;**7**:12207. DOI: 10.1038/ncomms12207

[32] Jiang S, Li C, Olive V, Lykken E, Feng F, Sevilla J, et al. Molecular dissection of the miR-17-92 cluster's critical dual roles in promoting Th1 responses and preventing inducible Treg differentiation. Blood. 2011;**118**(20):5487-5497. DOI: 10.1182/blood-2011-05-355644

[33] Smith KM, Guerau-de-Arellano M, Costinean S, Williams JL, Bottoni A, Mavrikis Cox G, et al. miR-29ab1 deficiency identifies a negative feedback loop controlling Th1 bias that is dysregulated in multiple sclerosis. Journal of Immunology. 2012;**189**(4):1567-1576. DOI: 10.4049/jimmunol.1103171

[34] Sawant DV, Wu H, Kaplan MH, Dent AL. The Bcl6 target gene microRNA-21 promotes Th2 differentiation by a T cell intrinsic pathway. Molecular Immunology. 2013;**54**(3-4):435-442. DOI: 10.1016/j.molimm.2013.01.006

[35] Mattes J, Collison A, Plank M, Phipps S, Foster PS. Antagonism of microRNA-126 suppresses the effector function of TH2 cells and the development of allergic airways disease. Proceedings of the National Academy of Sciences of the United States of America. 2009;**106**(44):18704-18709. DOI: 10.1073/pnas.0905063106

[36] Crazzolara R, Bendall L. Emerging treatments in acute lymphoblastic leukemia. Current Cancer Drug Targets. 2009;**9**(1):19-31. DOI: 10.2174/156800909787314057

[37] Li W-y, X-m C, Xiong W, D-m G, Lu L, Li H-y. Detection of microvesicle miRNA expression in ALL subtypes and analysis of their functional roles. Journal of Huazhong University of Science and Technology [Medical Sciences]. 2014;**34**(5):640-645. DOI: 10.1007/s11596-014-1330-0

[38] Pradillo M, Santos JL. Genes involved in miRNA biogenesis affect meiosis and fertility. Chromosome Research. 2018;**26**:1-9. DOI: 10.1007/s10577-018-9588-x

[39] Oliveira JC, Scrideli CA, Brassesco MS, Morales AG, Pezuk JA, Queiroz RP, et al. Differential MiRNA expression in childhood acute lymphoblastic leukemia and association with clinical and biological features. Leukemia Research. 2012;**36**(3):293-298. DOI: 10.1016/j.leukres.2011.10.005

[40] Santos Almeida R, Costa e Silva M, Coutinho LL, Gomes RG, Pedrosa F, Massaro JD, et al. MicroRNA expression profiles discriminate childhood T-from B-acute lymphoblastic leukemia. Hematological Oncology. 2018;**0**(0):2567. DOI: 10.1002/hon.2567

[41] Fulci V, Colombo T, Chiaretti S, Messina M, Citarella F, Tavolaro S, et al. Characterization of B- and T-lineage acute lymphoblastic leukemia by integrated analysis of MicroRNA and mRNA expression profiles. Genes, Chromosomes and Cancer. 2009;**48**(12):1069-1082. DOI: 10.1002/gcc.20709

[42] Schotte D, Chau JCK, Sylvester G, Liu G, Chen C, van der Velden VHJ, et al. Identification of new microRNA genes and aberrant microRNA profiles in childhood acute lymphoblastic leukemia. Leukemia. 2008;**23**(2): 313-322. DOI: 10.1038/leu.2008.28

[43] Malik D, Kaul D, Chauhan N, Marwaha RK. miR-2909-mediated regulation of KLF4: A novel molecular mechanism for differentiating between B-cell and T-cell pediatric acute lymphoblastic leukemias. Molecular Cancer. 2014;**13**:175-190. DOI: 10.1186/1476-4598-13-175

[44] Mavrakis KJ, Van Der Meulen J, Wolfe AL, Liu X, Mets E, Taghon T, et al. A cooperative microRNA-tumor suppressor gene network in acute T-cell lymphoblastic leukemia (T-ALL). Nature Genetics. 2011;**43**(7):673-678. DOI: 10.1038/ng.858

[45] Cao J, Cai J, Huang D, Han Q, Chen Y, Yang Q, et al. miR-335 represents an independent prognostic marker in epithelial ovarian cancer. American Journal of Clinical Pathology. 2014;**141**(3):437-442. DOI: 10.1309/AJCPLYTZGB54ISZC

[46] Bousquet M, Harris MH, Zhou B, Lodish HF. MicroRNA miR-125b causes leukemia. Proceedings of the National Academy of Sciences of the United States of America. 2010;**107**(50):21558-21563. DOI: 10.1073/pnas.1016611107

[47] Labib HA, Elantouny NG, Ibrahim NF, Alnagar AA. Upregulation of microRNA-21 is a poor prognostic marker in patients with childhood B cell acute lymphoblastic leukemia. Hematology. 2017;**22**(7):392-397. DOI: 10.1080/10245332.2017.1292204

[48] Li XJ, Luo XQ, Han BW, Duan FT, Wei PP, Chen YQ. MicroRNA-100/99a, deregulated in acute lymphoblastic leukaemia, suppress proliferation and promote apoptosis by regulating the FKBP51 and IGF1R/mTOR signalling pathways. British Journal of Cancer. 2013;**109**(8):2189-2198. DOI: 10.1038/bjc.2013.562

[49] Nemes K, Csóka M, Nagy N, Márk Á, Váradi Z, Dankó T, et al. Expression of certain leukemia/lymphoma related microRNAs and its correlation with prognosis in childhood acute lymphoblastic leukemia. Pathology & Oncology Research. 2015;**21**(3):597-604. DOI: 10.1007/s12253-014-9861-z

[50] Gefen N, Binder V, Zaliova M, Linka Y, Morrow M, Novosel A, et al. Hsa-mir-125b-2 is highly expressed in childhood ETV6/RUNX1 (TEL/AML1) leukemias and confers survival advantage to growth inhibitory signals independent of p53. Leukemia. 2010;**24**(1):89-96. DOI: 10.1038/leu.2009.208

[51] Ohyashiki JH, Umezu T, Kobayashi C, Hamamura RS, Tanaka M, Kuroda M, et al. Impact on cell to plasma ratio of miR-92a in patients with acute leukemia: in vivo assessment of cell to plasma ratio of miR-92a. BMC Research Notes. 2010;**3**:347. DOI: 10.1186/1756-0500-3-347

[52] Organista-Nava J, Gómez-Gómez Y, Illades-Aguiar B, Del Carmen Alarcón-Romero L, Saavedra-Herrera MV, Rivera-Ramírez AB, et al. High miR-24 expression is associated with risk of relapse and poor survival in acute leukemia. Oncology Reports. 2015;**33**(4):1639-1649. DOI: 10.3892/or.2015.3787

[53] Sugita F, Maki K, Nakamura Y, Sasaki K, Mitani K. Overexpression of MIR9 indicates poor prognosis in acute lymphoblastic leukemia. Leukemia & Lymphoma. 2014;**55**(1):78-86. DOI: 10.3109/10428194.2013.790023

[54] Wang Y, Li Z, He C, Wang D, Yuan X, Chen J, et al. MicroRNAs expression signatures are associated with lineage and survival in acute leukemias.

Blood Cells, Molecules & Diseases. 2010;**44**(3):191-197. DOI: 10.1016/j.bcmd.2009.12.010

[55] Mosakhani N, Sarhadi VK, Usvasalo A, Karjalainen-Lindsberg M-L, Lahti L, Tuononen K, et al. MicroRNA profiling in pediatric acute lymphoblastic leukemia: Novel prognostic tools. Leukemia & Lymphoma. 2012;**53**(12):2517-2520. DOI: 10.3109/10428194.2012.685731

[56] Yan J, Jiang N, Huang G, Tay JLS, Lin B, Bi C, et al. Deregulated MIR 335 that targets MAPK 1 is implicated in poor outcome of paediatric acute lymphoblastic leukaemia. British Journal of Haematology. 2013;**163**(1): 93-103. DOI: 10.1111/bjh.12489

[57] Piatopoulou D, Avgeris M, Drakaki I, Marmarinos A, Xagorari M, Baka M, et al. Clinical utility of miR-143/miR-182 levels in prognosis and risk stratification specificity of BFM-treated childhood acute lymphoblastic leukemia. Annals of Hematology. 2018;**97**(7):1169-1182. DOI: 10.1007/s00277-018-3292-y

[58] Mei Y-Y, Li Z-G, Zhang Y, Zhang W-L, Zhang P-W, Wang N, et al. Prognostic significance of joint detection of miR-210 and minimal residual disease in pediatric acute lymphoblastic leukemia. Zhongguo Shi Yan Xue Ye Xue Za Zhi. 2017;**25**(1):66-71. DOI: 10.7534/j.issn.1009-2137.2017.01.011

[59] Mei Y, Gao C, Wang K, Cui L, Li W, Zhao X, et al. Effect of microRNA-210 on prognosis and response to chemotherapeutic drugs in pediatric acute lymphoblastic leukemia. Cancer Science. 2014;**105**(4):463-472. DOI: 10.1111/cas.12370

[60] Zhou G, Cao Y, Dong W, Lin Y, Wang Q, Wu W, et al. The clinical characteristics and prognostic significance of AID, miR-181b, and miR-155 expression in adult patients with de novo B-cell acute lymphoblastic leukemia. Leukemia & Lymphoma. 2017;**58**(9):2118-2126. DOI: 10.1080/10428194.2017.1283028

[61] Xu L, Y-n L, X-q L, X-d L, H-x G. Association of miRNAs expression profiles with prognosis and relapse in childhood acute lymphoblastic leukemia. Zhonghua Xue Ye Xue Za Zhi. 2011;**32**(3):178-181

[62] Kaddar T, Chien WW, Bertrand Y, Pages MP, Rouault JP, Salles G, et al. Prognostic value of miR-16 expression in childhood acute lymphoblastic leukemia relationships to normal and malignant lymphocyte proliferation. Leukemia Research. 2009;**33**(9):1217-1223. DOI: 10.1016/j.leukres.2008.12.015

[63] Tong L-G, Wu W-Z, Zhang Y-P, Zhou Z-G, Chen Y-F, Huang W-J, et al. Expression of miR-16 in patients with T lymphoblastic lymphoma/acute lymphoblastic leukemia. Zhongguo Shi Yan Xue Ye Xue Za Zhi. 2014;**22**(1):99-103. DOI: 10.7534/j.issn.1009-2137.2014.01.020

[64] Li J, Li P, Wang J, Xi Y. Significance of microRNA-16 and bcl-2 expression in T lymphoblastic lymphoma/leukemia and its relation with prognosis. Zhonghua Bing Li Xue Za Zhi. 2013;**42**(11):748-752. DOI: 10.3760/cma.j.issn.0529-5807.2013.11.007

[65] Gimenes-Teixeira HL, Lucena-Araujo AR, Dos Santos GA, Zanette DL, Scheucher PS, Oliveira LC, et al. Increased expression of miR-221 is associated with shorter overall survival in T-cell acute lymphoid leukemia. Experimental Hematology & Oncology. 2013;**2**(1):10. DOI: 10.1186/2162-3619-2-10

[66] Oliveira LH, Schiavinato JL, Fráguas MS, Lucena-Araujo AR, Haddad R, Araújo AG, et al. Potential roles of microRNA-29a in the molecular

pathophysiology of T-cell acute lymphoblastic leukemia. Cancer Science. 2015;**106**(10):1264-1277. DOI: 10.1111/cas.12766

[67] Schaaf MJM, Cidlowski JA. Molecular mechanisms of glucocorticoid action and resistance. The Journal of Steroid Biochemistry and Molecular Biology. 2002;**83**(1):37-48. DOI: 10.1016/S0960-0760(02)00263-7

[68] Xu L, Liang Y, Luo X, Liu X, Guo H. Association of miRNAs expression profiles with prognosis and relapse in childhood acute lymphoblastic leukemia. Zhonghua xue ye xue za zhi= Zhonghua xueyexue zazhi. 2011;**32**(3):178-181

[69] Schotte D, De Menezes RX, Akbari Moqadam F, Khankahdani LM, Lange-Turenhout E, Chen C, et al. MicroRNA characterize genetic diversity and drug resistance in pediatric acute lymphoblastic leukemia. Haematologica. 2011;**96**(5):703-711. DOI: 10.3324/haematol.2010.026138

[70] Pui CH, Chessells JM, Camitta B, Baruchel A, Biondi A, Boyett JM, et al. Clinical heterogeneity in childhood acute lymphoblastic leukemia with 11q23 rearrangements. Leukemia. 2003;**17**(4):700-706. DOI: 10.1038/sj.leu.2402883

[71] Kotani A, Ha D, Hsieh J, Rao PK, Schotte D, den Boer ML, et al. miR-128b is a potent glucocorticoid sensitizer in MLL-AF4 acute lymphocytic leukemia cells and exerts cooperative effects with miR-221. Blood. 2009;**114**(19):4169-4178. DOI: 10.1182/blood-2008-12-191619

[72] Kotani A, Ha D, Schotte D, den Boer ML, Armstrong SA, Lodish HF. A novel mutation in the miR-128b gene reduces miRNA processing and leads to glucocorticoid resistance of MLL-AF4 acute lymphocytic leukemia cells. Cell cycle (Georgetown, Tex). 2010;**9**(6):1037-1042. DOI: 10.4161/cc.9.6.11011

[73] Shah MY, Ferrajoli A, Sood AK, Lopez-Berestein G, Calin GA. microRNA therapeutics in cancer—An emerging concept. eBioMedicine. 2016;**12**:34-42. DOI: 10.1016/j.ebiom.2016.09.017

[74] Nishioka C, Ikezoe T, Yang J, Nobumoto A, Tsuda M, Yokoyama A. Downregulation of miR-217 correlates with resistance of Ph(+) leukemia cells to ABL tyrosine kinase inhibitors. Cancer Science. 2014;**105**(3):297-307. DOI: 10.1111/cas.12339

[75] Bueno MJ, de Castro IP, de Cedrón MG, Santos J, Calin GA, Cigudosa JC, et al. Genetic and epigenetic silencing of microRNA-203 enhances ABL1 and BCR-ABL1 oncogene expression. Cancer Cell. 2016;**29**(4):607-608. DOI. 10.1016/j.ccell.2016.03.013

[76] Dou L, Zheng D, Li J, Li Y, Gao L, Wang L, et al. Methylation-mediated repression of microRNA-143 enhances MLL–AF4 oncogene expression. Oncogene. 2011;**31**(4):507-517. DOI: 10.1038/onc.2011.248

[77] Pineau P, Volinia S, McJunkin K, Marchio A, Battiston C, Terris B, et al. miR-221 overexpression contributes to liver tumorigenesis. Proceedings of the National Academy of Sciences of the United States of America. 2010;**107**(1):264-269. DOI: 10.1073/pnas.0907904107

[78] Felli N, Fontana L, Pelosi E, Botta R, Bonci D, Facchiano F, et al. MicroRNAs 221 and 222 inhibit normal erythropoiesis and erythroleukemic cell growth via kit receptor down-modulation. Proceedings of the National Academy of Sciences of the United States of America. 2005;**102**(50):18081-18086. DOI: 10.1073/pnas.0506216102

Chapter 5

New Protein Markers of Chronic Lymphocytic and Acute Lymphocytic Leukemia

Martina Maďarová, Dominik Dobransky and Tomas Dobransky

Abstract

There is an urgent need for the application of new protein markers in early and personalized prognostic diagnosis of cancer. As with many other types of malignancies, the number of leukemia-affected patients is on the rise. This requires novel tools when it comes to efficient treatment approaches, specifically those that are preventative and highly precise. Numerous important discoveries have recently been published regarding new proteins and their pathology-related modifications, which may play important roles in the onset and progression of leukemia. Chronic and acute lymphocytic leukemia are represented by important changes in lymphocyte cell metabolism, where many of the regulating transmembrane protein markers demonstrate altered functions in the regulation of crucial cell transduction signaling pathways. The most notable progress thus far has been achieved in studies concerning CD5, CD10, CD19, CD20, CD22, CD23, and CD52 protein markers and their associated proteins. As such, some of these signals may be applied in specific and personalized diagnostics as well as drug development.

Keywords: chronic lymphocytic leukemia, acute lymphocytic leukemia, protein markers, disease proteomics, personalized cancer diagnosis

1. Introduction

Chronic lymphocytic leukemia (CLL) is the most common malignancy in adults, and acute lymphocytic leukemia (ALL) is the most common pediatric cancer in western countries. These leukemic diseases affect the lymphoid line of blood cells. In most cases, the cause is unknown, hypothesizing that multiple genetic mutations and epigenetic changes are involved. Both diseases are vastly heterogeneous. While CLL is generally considered incurable and progresses slowly in most cases, ALL progresses rapidly and is typically fatal within weeks or months if left untreated. Historically, survival rates have been poor for patients with ALL. Since the introduction of chemotherapy, prognosis for childhood leukemia has improved greatly, and children with ALL are estimated to have a 95% probability of achieving successful remission. However, a total of 10–15% of patients still relapse despite undergoing intensive chemotherapy, and outcomes are far less encouraging in adults. CLL treatment tends to focus mainly on controlling the state of the disease and its associated symptoms, rather than on its definitive eradication. The specifics of treatment will largely depend on the patient's prognosis and the specific CLL subtype. Therefore, lifelong observation and follow-up are strongly recommended and supported for all the patients. The combination of chemotherapy and non-chemotherapeutic drugs has improved survival of CLL patients overall, leading to long-lasting remissions. The pathology of CLL is complex in that it is influenced by a number of genetic and molecular changes, the CLL microenvironment, as well as various signaling pathways, of which the B-cell receptor (BCR) signaling pathway is central to CLL activation. Signaling pathways that are identified as being affected in CLL patients can provide opportunities for the development of disease-specific drugs to the extent that they may be applicable in future clinical testing and molecular treatments. In any type of cancer, molecular therapy which targets specific regulatory proteins or their disease-associated posttranslational modifications can make way for novel applications which provide even higher specificity and efficiency with regard to treatment. This approach certainly applies to any type of leukemia.

2. Chronic lymphocytic leukemia

Chronic lymphocytic leukemia (CLL) is the most prevalent adult leukemia in the western world. The disease typically occurs in elderly patients and has a highly variable clinical progression. CLL is characterized by the clonal expansion and accumulation of mature CD19+, CD5+, and CD23+ B lymphocytes in the peripheral blood, bone marrow, and secondary lymphoid organs [1]. CLL cells are phenotypically similar to antigen-experienced B cells and show gene expression profiles similar to memory B cells [2]. The cellular origin of CLL is still debated, but it is assumed that CLL cells originate either from unmutated mature CD5+ B cells or CD5+CD27+ post-germinal center B-cell subsets [3]. CLL cells recirculate between peripheral blood and secondary lymphoid organs, where they proliferate in distinct areas of tissue, termed "pseudofollicles," at a daily birth rate of approximately 1–2% of the entire clone size [4]. Survival of CLL cells strictly depends on a permissive microenvironment composed of cellular components such as monocyte-derived nurse-like cells, T cells, follicular dendritic cells, mesenchymal stromal cells, and endothelial cells. Such dynamic combination of components leads to the presence of molecules such as cytokines, chemokines, and angiogenic factors. Leukemic cells take advantage of these vital proteins by interacting with them via cell-surface receptors or cell adhesion molecules to further facilitate their proliferation and survival [5, 6]. CLL cells are also characterized by an often observed defect in apoptosis which allows peripheral blood B lymphocytes to survive [7].

Autoantigens and/or autonomous mechanisms activate the BCR and its signaling cascade in secondary lymphatic tissues, playing a central pathogenic role in CLL [8]. These events result in activation of multiple downstream regulators in B cells which ultimately mediate changes in cell proliferation, survival, and migration via both transcriptional modulation and phosphorylation. BCR signaling responses in CLL cells are heterogeneous, with effective activation of only a selected set of downstream responses [9]. Another key property of BCRs is that they exhibit somatic mutations in varying amounts; importantly, the degree of mutation has been found to inform the prognosis of disease [2, 10]. Furthermore, many cases of CLL (approximately one third) are characterized by a nearly indistinguishable subset of BCRs exhibiting shared antigens. This suggests a close link between these specific molecules and CLL pathogenesis.

CLL cells usually show constitutive phosphorylation of signaling proteins which promote their proliferation and survival, leading to pathological processes. Protein phosphorylation in lymphocytes is tightly associated with the regulation of a variety of protein activities, functional regulation, and cell signaling and may thus affect initiation and/or progression of the disease. As such, protein phosphorylation may be one of the most promising targets for the discovery of novel cancer-related protein markers and in turn their application in new approaches to molecular therapy. The constitutive activation of proteins by phosphorylation presents its potential for prognostic significance, as the identification of aberrant signal transduction in leukemic cells can become a potential target for novel agents. After BCR stimulation, CLL cells have shown a tendency toward impaired phosphorylation levels. Higher basal phosphorylation levels of PLCγ2 (pY759), p44/42 MAPK (pT202/Y204), p38 MAPK (pT180/Y182), NF-κB p65 (pS529), STAT5 (pY694), and STAT6 (pY641) were detected in CLL cells compared to normal B cells, predicting their impaired function [12]. As such, these markers may represent some of the novel protein targets involved in the development of efficient therapeutics. Cancer cells with constitutive STAT3 activation have been reported to have elevated levels of cell cycle regulation and antiapoptotic proteins, leading to apoptotic resistance. Constitutive serine phosphorylation of STAT1 and STAT3 has also been reported in CLL cells [13]. More recently, new phosphorylations on threonine (pThr314) and two serine residues (pSer254, pSer265) of CD23, which is overexpressed and abnormally regulated in CLL, were reported in B lymphocytes of B-CLL patients [14]. Regulation of these CD23, CLL-associated phosphorylation sites brings new insight to the involvement of this transmembrane protein marker in the onset and progress of CLL.

2.1 Incidence and risk

CLL is the most common leukemia in western countries, with an estimated incidence of about 4.5 new cases per 100,000 individuals annually [1]. It is most frequent in white populations in the United States and the lowest in Eastern Asian populations [15]. Median age at diagnosis is usually 72 years, and more male than female patients (1.7:1) are affected. About 10% of CLL patients are reported to be younger than 55 years of age [16].

The etiology of CLL is still unknown. Genetics and environmental factors may play an important role. Over 25 gene polymorphisms have been identified as contributing to CLL from a familial standpoint. These include genes that play roles in apoptosis, B-cell biology, as well as regulation by microRNAs, all of which have been found to be involved in disease progression [17, 18]. As such, it is important to note that relative to the general population, a six- to ninefold greater risk of developing the disease exists in individuals who have or have had relatives with CLL. Consequent protein synthesis and the involvement of newly synthesized proteins in disease onset and progression are the focus of numerous current studies. Insecticide exposure and farming history have also been associated with a higher environmental risk for developing CLL [19].

2.2 Symptoms and diagnosis

According to the International Workshop on Chronic Lymphocytic Leukemia (iwCLL) 2008 guidelines [20], a CLL diagnosis is established by the presence of more than 5×10^9/L peripheral lymphocytes, which lasts for a duration of at least 3 months, co-expressing CD5-, CD19-, and CD23-positive and weakly expressing CD20- and CD79b-positive as well as surface immunoglobulins.

Immunophenotyping by flow cytometry is required to establish CLL diagnosis based on cell identity, clonality, and quantity [21].

Two clinical staging systems, the Rai et al. [22] and Binet et al. [23] systems, are used to group patients with CLL into risk groups with discrete clinical outcomes. These two staging systems are relatively simple and widely used, relying on a physical examination and standard laboratory tests. Notably, the clinical presentation of CLL at diagnosis is extremely variable. Approximately 60% of patients are asymptomatic, and it is possible to detect the presence of the disease via a routine blood cell count. Lymphadenopathy (80%) and splenomegaly (50%) may be observed. Hepatomegaly is less frequent. As the disease progresses, patients can have B symptoms (weight loss, fever, night sweats, weakness) and exhibit a higher risk of infections. Lymphocytosis is constantly present, but the absolute number of lymphocytes is extremely variable. Anemia and thrombocytopenia may be also observed in 15–30% of patients [22–24]. Monoclonal B lymphocytosis (MBL), which can be observed in 5% of patients who exhibit a regular blood count and no other characteristics of a lymphoproliferative disposition, is characterized by a monoclonal B lymphocyte number of less than 5×10^9/L in circulating blood [25]. Advancement from MBL to CLL is seen in a frequency of 1–2% cases per year [26].

Small lymphocytic lymphoma (SLL), in which the same leukemic cell population is mostly restricted to the bone marrow and lymphoid tissues, is similarly managed but considered to be a single entity [27]. The transformation into Richter syndrome (most commonly diffuse large B-cell lymphoma) occurs in 5–10% of all CLL cases and usually has a very poor prognosis [16].

2.3 Prognostic factors

The most important prognostic factors aside from clinical Rai and Binet staging systems are serum markers including β2 microglobulin levels [28], thymidine kinase levels [29], soluble CD23 levels [30], cellular markers including CD38 [31] and ζ chain associated protein kinase 70 (ZAP70) [32], CD49d [33], chemokines CCL3 a CCL4, genetic parameters including the mutational status of IGHV genes [10], and cytogenetic aberrations [34]. Unfavorable prognostic factors also include the male gender, ≥65 years of age, poor performance status due to medical comorbidities, late-stage disease at diagnosis, an initial white blood cell count above 35×10^9/L, lymphocyte doubling time of less than 6 months, and a diffuse histological pattern in bone marrow infiltration [35]. Elevated levels of beta-2 microglobulin, serum thymidine, and serum CD23 at diagnosis also result in a poor prognosis [36].

ZAP-70 is a cytoplasmic protein tyrosine kinase initially identified in T cells. ZAP-70 expression in CLL is associated with increased BCR signaling capacity and greater responsiveness to chemokines resulting in more pronounced CLL cell migration and activation. Patients with ZAP-70 expression in more than 20% of CLL cells have a relatively shorter median time from diagnosis to initial treatment [37], and ZAP-70 appears to be a risk factor that is closely linked to aggressive CLL [32]. CD38 is a transmembrane protein that supports B-cell interaction and differentiation through the binding of CD31 [38], a cell adhesion molecule expressed by cells of the CLL microenvironment. Patients with high CD38 expression experience faster progression and shorter life expectancy [31]. The expression of the surface molecule CD49d, the α4 subunit of the integrin heterodimer α4β1, promotes microenvironment-mediated proliferation of CLL leukemic cells and has been identified in a subgroup of patients characterized by progression of disease and short survival [33]. Both CCL3 and CCL4 are members of a cluster of cytokines with function as chemoattractants for monocytes and lymphocytes. They promote the communication of survival and proliferation signals to malignant cells and are associated with worse clinical outcomes in CLL [39, 40].

Immunoglobulin heavy-chain variable region (IGHV) mutation status plays an important role in CLL prognosis. Based on the degree of somatic hypermutation IGHV segments, unmutated IGHV (98% or more sequence homology with the germline sequence) corresponds to CLL originating from B cells that have not undergone a somatic mutation. Such patients can be classified as "unmutated" (U-CLL). Mutated IGHV (less than 98% sequence homology) is referred to as "mutated" (M-CLL) cases [41]. The presence of unmutated IGHV predicts a more aggressive disease type and has traditionally been associated with significantly decreased survival rates compared with mutated IGHV, which is associated with slower disease progression and longer survival [10, 31]. The differences in clinical behavior between M-CLL and U-CLL are determined by differences in responsiveness to external signals (such as BCR responsiveness). U-CLL BCRs are polyreactive and mostly recognize autoantigens and other environmental antigens [42, 43]. In contrast, affinity-matured BCRs from M-CLL cases bind to a restricted set of more specific antigens that either occur infrequently or induce anergy. Consequently, the M-CLL clone remains stable overall or expands at a slower rate [44, 45].

More than 80% of patients with previously untreated CLL have cytogenetic abnormalities, most common of which is a deletion in chromosome del(13q) [del(13q14.1)] (55%), followed by del(11q) [del(11q22 23)] (10–25%), trisomy 12 (10–20%), and del(17p) [del(17p13)] (5–10%) [34, 46]. Recommended analyses include interphase cytogenetic analysis with FISH for the detection of the del(17p), which affects p53 expression. A positive outcome is often seen in individuals who have deletions in 13q. This is likely a result of two missing miRNAs typically found in 13q, miR-15-1, and miR-16-1, which exhibit strong activity in healthy B cells; miR-15-1 and miR-16-1 are thought to play a role in the downregulation of B-cell lymphoma 2 (BCL2), which acts as an antiapoptotic molecule [34].

The association between trisomy 12 and prognosis is still not clear [47]. A deletion in 11q results in the ataxia telangiectasia mutated (ATM) gene, which has shown to be a predictor of poor clinical outcome [34]. Deletions of the short arm of chromosome 17 cause the loss of one tumor protein p53 (TP53) allele and are associated with inactivating mutations in the other allele in 80% of patients with CLL. This cytogenetic aberration is associated with the worst CLL prognosis. Patients have shown marked resistance against genotoxic chemotherapies which has forced clinicians to alter their first-line treatment [34, 48]. Further recurring gene alterations have been found in 5% of cases of CLL samples at time of diagnosis; via whole genome/exome sequencing, genes influencing NOTCH1 and myeloid differentiation primary response (MYD88) [49] have been identified alongside genes coding for splicing factor 3B subunit 1 (SF3B1) [50] and baculoviral IAP repeat containing 3 (BIRC3) [51]. Patients experiencing progressive/refractory CLL and Richter's syndrome were observed to exhibit these mutations in greater frequency [50].

2.4 Therapy

CLL is an incurable disease with a highly heterogeneous clinical course. Previous studies have shown that early treatment with chemotherapeutic agents was unable to demonstrate a benefit due to these therapeutic interventions in CLL patients [52]. The standard treatment for patients with early disease is a "watch-and-wait" strategy. Treatment should only be initiated in patients with progressive or symptomatic/active disease. In order to determine the best approach to treatment, crucial factors such as the stage of disease, physical status, and cytogenetic risk should be assessed on a per-patient basis [18]. Additionally, the "Go-Go," "Slow-Go," and "No-Go" comorbidity classifications present another important set of factors in determining the optimal avenue for treatment [53].

Monotherapy with alkylating agents (chlorambucil) and purine analogs (fludarabine, pentostatin, cladribine, bendamustine) has served as an initial, frontline therapy for CLL and was the therapeutic "gold standard" for several decades [52]. Compared to monotherapy, the combination of fludarabine with alkylating cyclophosphamide is more widely used, leading to an increased effect on malignant lymphocytes and greater remission inductions [54]. The onset of biological treatment using monoclonal antibodies has led to significant changes in the approach to treatment. As CD20 is expressed on most B-cell malignancies, the introduction of the anti-CD20 antibody rituximab improved the treatment of most CD20-positive non-Hodgkin lymphomas, including CLL. Rituximab is less active as a single agent; however, combinations of rituximab with chemotherapy have shown to be very efficacious therapies for CLL [55]. The combination of rituximab, fludarabine, and cyclophosphamide is considered to be the standard first-line therapy (FCR chemoimmunotherapy) [56]. Ofatumumab and obinutuzumab are another set of CD20 antibodies used for the treatment of patients with relapsed/refractory CLL [57, 58]. Alemtuzumab is a recombinant, fully humanized, monoclonal antibody against the CD52 antigen. Monotherapy with alemtuzumab is used in patients with advanced CLL or relapsed patients after second-line fludarabine therapy and with poor prognostic features [59]. Autologous stem-cell transplantation is not useful in CLL. Maintenance therapy in CLL patients with higher risk of relapse may have some benefit but is not generally recommended [18].

Lenalidomide is an immunomodulatory agent that induces only mild apoptosis of leukemic cells but also reduces CLL proliferation through a cereblon-/p21-dependent mechanism. Lenalidomide has pleiotropic effects on the CLL microenvironment: it increases CD4+ T-mediated antigen presentation, proliferation, and activity and enhances NK and CD4+ T-cell mediated antitumor immune responses [60]. It is active alone, in CLL relapsed/refractory patients, or as an initial treatment for elderly patients or in combination with rituximab [61].

The CXCR4/CXCL12 signaling axis represents another important therapeutic target in CLL. CXCR4 antagonists have been developed, including peptide CXCR4 antagonists (BKT140), small molecule CXCR4 antagonists (AMD3100, plerixafor), and antibodies to CXCR4 (MDX-1338) [62]. Plerixafor inhibits CXCL12-mediated signaling activation on CLL cells and is used in combination with rituximab in relapsed CLL patients [63].

Proteins in the Bcl-2 family are key regulators of the apoptotic process with proapoptotic and prosurvival activities. Venetoclax is a so-called BH3-mimetic drug designed to block the function of the Bcl-2 protein and inhibits the growth of BCL-2-dependent tumors in vivo. Monotherapy with this drug is active and well tolerated in patients with relapsed or refractory del(17p) CLL, providing a new therapeutic option for this very poor prognosis population [64].

B-cell receptor signaling seems to play an important role in the survival of CLL cells. Inhibitors targeting BCR-associated kinases have changed the landscape of treatment for CLL patients, inducing durable remissions in relapsed/refractory patients, including those carrying unfavorable genetic alterations (e.g., del17p, del11q) [65]. Randomized trials comparing new drugs and/or their combinations with standard chemoimmunotherapy regimens are ongoing and will allow to better define optimal treatment strategies [66]. New light shed onto the mechanisms of BCR activation in CLL has enabled for the design and application of kinase inhibitors targeting BCR signaling kinases BTK, PI3K, and SYK. Bruton's tyrosine kinase, BTK, is a non-receptor tyrosine kinase that plays a central role in downstream activation of cell survival pathways such as NF-κB and MAP kinases via Src family kinases. Ibrutinib is the first human BTK inhibitor. The drug binds irreversibly to a cysteine residue (Cys-481) in the BTK kinase domain [67] and inhibits BTK phosphorylation and its enzymatic activity [68]. Ibrutinib inhibits CLL cell survival and proliferation, as well as leukemia cell migration toward the tissue homing chemokines [69]. Previous tests have shown that ibrutinib yielded durable remissions in CLL/SLL patients with relapsed, refractory, or high-risk disease and in previously untreated older patients [70]. Acalabrutinib, a potentially more selective, irreversible BTK inhibitor has been tested and is currently under early clinical development [71]. PI3Kδ is expressed by hematopoietic cells and plays a critical role in B-cell homeostasis and function. Idelalisib is a highly selective PI3Kδ inhibitor, which antagonizes CLL-survival signals coming from the microenvironment as well as BCR stimulation [72]. This drug inhibits CLL cell chemotaxis toward CXCL12 and CXCL13 and migration beneath stromal cells and also inhibits BCR- and chemokine-receptor-induced AKT and MAP kinase activation [73]. Idelalisib has been tested as single agent or in combination strategies with clinical benefit in patients with relapsed/refractory CLL [74]. Additional PI3K inhibitors are currently under development, including duvelisib, a potent PI3K γδ inhibitor, which antagonizes BCR and microenvironment interactions in vitro [75]. Spleen tyrosine kinase (SYK), which belongs to the SYK/ZAP70 family of non-receptor kinases, has been implicated in tissue homing and retention of activated B cells due to its role as a downstream activator of BCR signaling (chemokine and integrin receptors) [76]. Up to this point, only limited responses have been seen in patients experiencing CLL relapse after introduction of fostamatinib disodium (FosD) to the treatment regimen [77]. FosD is currently the only available inhibitor of SYK on the market, with additional similar drugs being developed [78].

3. Acute lymphocytic leukemia

Acute lymphocytic leukemia (ALL), also known as acute lymphoblastic leukemia or acute lymphoid leukemia, is the most common malignancy in children and the least common type of leukemia in adults. It is an acute type of cancer invading blood and spreading throughout the body to other organs, such as the liver, spleen, lymph nodes, and central nervous system. Without treatment, it can be fatal within a few months. ALL is characterized by a malignant transformation and proliferation of lymphoid progenitor cells in the bone marrow, blood, and extramedullary sites, which replace normal blood cells [79]. The exact causes of ALL remain largely unknown, but it is thought to result from genetic alterations such as structural chromosome rearrangements, aneuploidy, and mutations in genes that encode for transcription factors regulating lymphoid development, tumor suppressors, proteins that regulate cell cycle progression, and epigenetic modifiers. Such defects result in abnormal growth [80].

3.1 Classification

ALL is a hematologic malignancy with uncontrolled proliferation of lymphoblasts of B- or T-cell origin. ALL cases are clinically classified as B-cell precursor (BCP), mature B-cell, or T-cell types. BCP-ALL arises in B lymphocytes in the early stages of development in the bone marrow and affects 75–80% of adult patients. Mature B-cell ALL arises in more mature developing lymphocytes. This type of ALL is less common and accounts for around 3–5% of all adult cases. In around 20–25% of cases, ALL arises in developing T cells. This type of ALL can be further classified as early, mid, or late, depending on the maturity of the affected cell. T-cell ALL is commonly presented with a high white blood cell count and involvement of the central nervous system at diagnosis [81] (**Table 1**).

3.2 Incidence and risk

The incidence of ALL is estimated at 1.7 per 100,000 population in the United States [82] and 1.28 per 1 000,000 individuals in Europe [83] each year. ALL is the most frequent cancer in children, accounting for 30% of all cancers and 80% of leukemias, with peak incidence occurring at 2–5 years of age. The incidence decreases with age progression and rises back up with a second peak in patients above the age of 50 years, representing about 15% of leukemias [84]. ALL is more common in males than females. Survival rates were poor 50 years ago, when leukemia was considered to be an intractable disease. Currently, pediatric patients with ALL have dramatic cure rates with 80–90% achieving complete remission (CR) [85]. However, prognoses in the elderly remain miserable. Despite a high rate of response to induction chemotherapy, only 30–40% of adult patients with ALL will achieve long-term remission [86].

There are a few risk factors which can increase the possibility for ALL, such as exposure to high levels of radiation, industrial chemicals (such as benzene), pesticides [87], certain types of chemotherapy used to treat other cancers, certain types of viral infections (human T-cell lymphoma/leukemia virus-1 or Epstein-Barr virus) [88], inherited genetic syndromes (such as Down syndrome) [89], and being white and male.

3.3 Symptoms and diagnosis

Most clinical manifestations of ALL exhibit the accumulation of malignant, poorly differentiated lymphoid cells within the bone marrow, peripheral blood, and other tissues. Symptoms of ALL are generally nonspecific with a combination of constitutional symptoms and signs of bone marrow failure (anemia, thrombocytopenia, leukopenia). Common symptoms include "B symptoms"

ALL classification	Subtypes	Ref
B-ALL	B-cell precursor ALL (75–80%)	[81]
	Mature B-cell ALL (3–5%)	
T-ALL	Early T-cell precursor ALL (20%)	
	Mid or late subtypes of T-ALL (5%)	

Table 1.
Classification of ALL subtypes.

(fever, weight loss, night sweats), easy bruising or bleeding, fatigue, dyspnea, and infections. Lymphadenopathy, splenomegaly, or hepatomegaly can be also present [90, 91]. CNS involvement at time of diagnosis occurs in 5–8% of patients and presents most commonly as cranial nerve deficits or meningismus [86]. Current standards for the diagnosis of ALL are based on the classification of lymphoid neoplasms according to the World Health Organization (WHO) 2008 criterion [92]. Diagnosis of ALL is established by the presence of 20% or more lymphoblasts in the bone marrow or peripheral blood [90]. Flow cytometry and cytogenetic testing are needed to confirm the diagnosis and provide risk stratification. Immunophenotyping by flow cytometry has become the standard procedure for ALL diagnosis and subclassification and was also developed as a useful tool for the detection and monitoring of minimal residual disease. In B-lineage ALL, the most important markers for diagnosis, differential diagnosis, and subclassification are CD19, CD10, CD20, CD22, CD24, and CD79a [93, 94]. For T-lineage, they are CD1a, CD2, CD3, CD4, CD5, CD7, and CD8 [95]. Cytogenetics and karyotyping are helpful in the identification of recurrent translocations, chromosomal abnormalities, and numerical alterations. Fluorescence in situ hybridization (FISH) is a useful technique for detecting and localizing the presence or absence of specific DNA sequences on chromosomes, with 99% sensitivity. Finally, array-comparative genomic hybridization (array-CGH, a-CGH) and single-nucleotide polymorphism (SNP) arrays can facilitate the identification of cryptic and/or submicroscopic changes in the genome [96, 97]. Lumbar puncture with CSF analysis is the current standard of care for the diagnosis of CNS involvement. If the CNS is involved, brain MRIs should be performed. Other possible evaluations include a complete blood count alongside cytologic analysis of target cells to evaluate other hematopoietic cell lines, coagulation profiles, and serum chemistries [80].

3.4 Prognostic factors

ALL is a highly heterogeneous disease, and several clinical and biologic characteristics of ALL are used in risk stratification and prognostication. Disease characteristics (e.g., cytogenetics, molecular genetics, immunophenotypes) are substantially different between childhood, young adult, and adult ALL cases. Prognostic factors applied to ALL include age, white blood cell count (WBC), time to achieve a complete hematologic remission, minimal residual disease (MRD) persistence [98], and genetic aberrations. Older age and higher leukocyte count are associated with poor prognosis. Children older than 10 years with a leukocyte count exceeding 50,000/mm^3 are classified as high risk according to the National Cancer Institute criteria (NCI-HR) [99]. ALL in young adults leads to poorer outcomes and exhibits high-risk genomic features (BCR-ABL1, BCR-ABL1-like, ETP-ALL [100], JAK mutation, CRLF2 alteration [101], iAMP21 [102], or DUX4 translocation [103]). The National Cancer Institute defined adolescent and young adults (AYA) to be those aged 15–39 years old. AYAs may benefit from pediatric-inspired regimens and are thus considered separate from adults >40 years [104]. Elderly patients tend to have a form of the disease characterized by intrinsically unfavorable biology (BCR-ABL1, BCR-ABL1-like, hypodiploidy, and complex karyotype), more medical comorbidities, and an inability to tolerate standard chemotherapies. They also experience a higher risk of relapse. As such, patients over the age of 60 have particularly poor outcomes, with only 10–15% surviving long term [105]. Response to chemotherapy is a strong prognostic indicator in ALL. Clearance of leukemic blasts in the early phase of treatment and the achievement of remission at the end of induction are predictors of relapse risk and have prognostic importance. Gender has also been recognized as a prognostic factor, with females having a better outcome than males overall.

3.4.1 Cytogenetic/genetic risk

Cytogenetic analyses have demonstrated that chromosomal aberrations (insertions, deletions, translocations, and inversions) and numerical alterations (hyperdiploid, pseudodiploid, and hypodiploid) are hallmarks of ALL [106]. The prevalence of genetic subtypes differs with age and is of prognostic relevance. Approximately half of pediatric leukemia cases involve aneuploidy (with changes in chromosome number), including high hyperdiploidy (50–67 chromosomes) or hypodiploidy (44 chromosomes or fewer) [107]. The chromosome most frequently gained in patients with high hyperdiploidy is 21 (>90% cases with trisomy or tetrasomy of chromosome 21) [108]. It is thought that the duplication of specific chromosomes contributes to leukemogenesis, making high hyperdiploidy a stronger prognostic factor than hypodiploidy. Hypodiploidy has been associated with dismal prognosis in all observed cases of ALL. Near-haploid (24–31 chromosomes) and low-hypodiploid (32–39 chromosomes) ALLs exhibit activation of Ras- and PI3K-signaling pathways, suggesting that these pathways may be a target for therapy in aggressive hypodiploid ALLs [109]. Studies in the pediatric population have identified genetic syndromes that are connected to the predisposition in a minority of cases of ALL, such as Down syndrome, Fanconi anemia, Bloom syndrome, ataxia telangiectasia, and Nijmegen breakdown syndrome [89, 110, 111].

Characteristic translocations include erythroblast transformation-specific (ETS) variant 6–Runt-related transcription factor 1 (ETV6-RUNX1), the most common translocation (15–25% of pediatric ALL patients) caused by t(12;21)(p13;q22). The prognosis of ALL with ETV6-RUNX1 is excellent [112]. A second common translocation in pediatric ALL is transcription factor 3-PBX homeobox 1 (TCF3-PBX1), which is caused by t(1;19)(q23;p13) and is observed in 5–10% of ALL cases. Previously, patients with this translocation were considered to have poor prognosis, but a recently improved treatment has resulted in better outcomes [113]. A small percentage of ALL patients (3–5%) exhibit the reciprocal translocation t(9;22)(q34;q11), also referred to as the "Philadelphia (Ph) chromosome." The Ph chromosome is largely prominent in patients suffering from chronic myeloid leukemia (CML) and is molecularly characterized by the creation of a non-receptor tyrosine kinase gene (BCR-ABL1) via the fusion of RhoGEF and GTPase-activating protein (BCR) and ABL proto-oncogene 1 (ABL1) [114].

The prevalence of t(9;22) in adult ALL can range from 15 to 50% and increases with age [115]. Ph chromosome positivity has been widely considered to be a factor for poor prognosis. The development of tyrosine kinase inhibitors (TKI), which directly target BCR-ABL1, has shown to significantly improve the treatment strategy for Ph-ALL. Rearrangement of the mixed-lineage leukemia 1 gene (MML1), also known as KMT2A (lysine [K]-specific methyltransferase 2A), on chromosome 11q23 is found in a unique group of acute leukemias and predicts a very poor outcome [116].

More recently, a variant with a similar gene expression profile to Ph-positive ALL, but without the BCR-ABL1 rearrangement, has been identified. This so-called Ph-like ALL, or BCR-ABL1-like ALL, has been associated with poor response to induction chemotherapy, elevated minimal residual disease, and poor survival [117]. The prevalence of Ph-like ALL is common among all ages, ranging from 10 to 15% in children to over 25% in young adults [118]. Patients with Ph-like ALL harbor a diverse range of genetic alterations which activate cytokine receptor and kinase signaling pathways. Common genomic features of Ph-like ALL include alterations of B-lymphoid transcription factor genes (particularly IKZF1 deletions) as well as rearrangements and mutations of CRLF2, ABL-class tyrosine kinase genes, EPOR, JAK-STAT signaling, and RAS signaling (NRAS, KRAS, PTPN11, NF1) and other less common kinase alterations (FLT3, NTRK3, BLNK, TYK2, PTK2B) [119]. These mutated genes can be successfully targeted with tyrosine kinase inhibitors [117]. Another new high-risk subtype identified in diagnosis of ALL is B-ALL, which is characterized by intrachromosomal amplification of chromosome 21 (iAMP21) [102].

Genome-wide profiling studies have revealed components of multiple cellular and signaling pathways that are frequently mutated in ALL (referred to as cooperative mutations). Deletions in key transcription factors involved in B-cell development include IKAROS family zinc finger 1 (IKZF1), transcription factor 3 (E2A), early B-cell factor 1 (EBF1), and paired box 5 (PAX5). Kinase-activating mutations include rearrangements involving ABL1, JAK2, PDGFRB, CRLF2 and EPOR, activating mutations of IL7R and FLT3, and deletion of SH2B3, as well as mutations involved in tumor suppression (CDKN2A/CDKN2B, PTEN, and RB1), RAS signaling (NRAS, KRAS, and PTPN11), transcriptional regulation (ETV6, ERG, TBL1XR1, and CREBBP), and epigenetic modification (CREBBP, EP300, SETD2, and NSD2) [117]. In all ALL subtypes, multiple cooperating mutations are acquired or enriched for during leukemia development and progression [120]. TP53 disruption has also been detected in relapsed B-ALL and T-ALL, as well as in newly diagnosed children and adult ALL cases. Correlation with poorer outcome has been illustrated and is associated with refractoriness to chemotherapy in adults [121].

Next-generation sequencing (NGS), most notably transcriptome sequencing, has led to the identification of several novel rearrangements that are not made evident by conventional genetic analysis, including DUX4-rearranged [122], MEF2D-rearranged [103], and ZNF384-rearranged B-ALL and ETV6-RUNX1-like B-ALL [123]. These new ALL subtypes have distinct clinical and biological characteristics. The prognosis of the B-ALL subtypes is shown in **Table 2**.

Molecular subtype	Prognosis	Frequency (%)	References
Hyperdiploid	Favorable	20–30	[107, 108]
ETV6-RUNX1	Favorable	15–25	[112]
TCF3-PBX1	Intermediate	5–10	[113]
KMT2A rearranged	Unfavorable	5	[116]
BCR-ABL1	Unfavorable	5–50	[114, 115]
BCR-ABL1 like	Unfavorable	10–25	[118]
Hypodiploid	Unfavorable	3	[109]
iAMP21	unfavorable	2	[102]
DUX4 rearranged	Favorable	4–5	[122]
MEF2D rearranged	Unfavorable	2–3	[103]
ZNF384 rearranged	Intermediate	2–3	[123]
ETV6-RUNX1 like	Intermediate	2–3	[123]

Favorable, intermediate, and unfavorable prognoses of acute lymphoblastic leukemia (ALL) subtypes are associated with 5-year overall survival of >90%, 70–90%, and <70%, respectively.

Table 2.
Prognosis in B-ALL.

T-ALL is characterized by numerous transcriptional, signaling, and epigenetic factors. Activating mutations in NOTCH1 can be found in the majority of T-ALL cases and predict a favorable prognosis [124]. Deletions of the CDKN2A locus encoding the P16/INK4A and P19/ARF tumor suppressors, responsible for control of cell cycle progression and P53 regulation, respectively, are present in about 70% of T-ALLs [125]. Gene expression profiling has identified major categories of T-ALL associated with gene expression during thymocyte development. Cytokine receptor RAS signaling genes, which include FLT3, have been found to be activated by mutation in early T-cell precursor T-ALL (ETP T-ALL). In addition, alterations in genes which disturb hematopoietic development, such as GATA 3, ETV6, and RUNX1, have been observed. Lastly, mutations in histone-modifying genes (EZH2, SUZ12, and EED) are also a consequence of ETP T-ALL. ETP T-ALL has been associated with poor prognosis [126]. Early cortical thymocyte leukemias are primarily associated with translocations resulting in aberrant expression of TLX1, TLX3, and related homeobox transcription factor oncogenes; these exhibit a characteristically favorable outcome [125, 127]. Late cortical leukemias occur further down in the pattern of gene expression programming related to T-cell development, overexpressing the transcription factor oncogene TAL1 with either LMO1 or LMO2 and PTEN. These are associated with poor prognosis [125, 127].

3.5 Therapy

Typical chemotherapy consists of induction, consolidation, and long-term maintenance, with CNS prophylaxis given at intervals throughout therapy. The goal of induction therapy is to achieve complete remission and to restore a normal blood cell count. Predominantly 85–90% of patients achieve complete remission after 4–6 weeks of this regimen [128]. Several chemotherapeutic agents are currently used in the treatment of CLL, including amascrine, asparaginase, cyclophosphamide, cytarabine, daunorubicin, dexamethasone, and methotrexate. Each utilizes slightly differing mechanisms of action; in the general sense however, these molecules affect the growth and division of cancer cells by inducing DNA damage [129]. Multi-agent cytotoxic chemotherapy has had great success in pediatric age groups [130]. Pediatric-inspired treatment protocols have also shown superior outcomes in young adults [104], but the same success has not been reproduced in adults despite regime modifications. Traditional adult treatment protocols include intensive myelosuppressive agents as well as allogeneic hematopoietic stem cell transplant (allo-SCT) in first remission [104]. After achieving complete response, treatment options include consolidation and maintenance chemotherapy or allo-SCT for eligible patients [131]. For high-risk patients (Ph-positive ALL, elevated WBC count, CNS disease, high-risk gene rearrangements, or hypodiploidy) and patients with relapsed/refractory disease, allo-SCT has long been considered the standard of care. However, the advent of TKIs marked a turning point in the treatment of some high-risk subtypes such as Ph-ALL and Ph-like ALL. After induction therapy, subsequent consolidation therapy begins to eradicate residual leukemic cells. Consolidation varies in different protocols but generally utilizes similar agents for induction (various combinations of cytotoxic agents and high dose of escalating methotrexate) and at times includes intrathecal chemotherapy and cranial radiation for CNS prophylaxis [132]. Maintenance therapy typically lasts 1–2 years. Daily 6-mercaptopurine (6-MP) and weekly MTX are a standard combination, and some maintenance therapies are enhanced with vincristine and steroids [80].

A better understanding of the molecular landscape of ALL and advances in the field of monoclonal antibody therapy have resulted in the development of several new agents, especially in the treatment of adolescent and young adults (AYA) and adult patients. Targeted delivery of monoclonal antibodies based on leukemic cell-surface receptor recognition improves efficacy and minimizes off-target toxicity. The antigens CD19, CD20, CD22, and CD52 are the most common antigens to which monoclonal antibodies in B-cell ALL have been directed. Rituximab is a non-conjugated monoclonal antibody designed to target a single antigen on the tumor cell surface. The combination of rituximab with chemotherapy in the frontline treatment of CD20-positive B-ALL has been shown to increase CR duration, lower relapse rates, and improve event-free survival [133]. A new generation of monoclonal antibodies exists which is characterized by the antibody being conjugated to drug or toxins with the purpose of enhancing the efficiency of cancer cell killing. For example, inotuzumab ozogamicin (IO) is a monoclonal antibody against CD22 linked to the cytotoxic agent, calicheamicin. The use of IO alone, and in combination with chemotherapy, has shown promise in relapsed and refractory B-cell ALL [134]. Other modifications to antibody constructs can also augment immunogenic reactions against leukemia. Blinatumomab is the first approved drug in the BiTE class, a bispecific T-cell receptor engager, which has both a monoclonal antibody against CD19 and an anti-CD3 T cell-binding domain. Monotherapy in relapsed and refractory B-cell ALL has resulted in prolonged relapse-free survival [135]. The effectiveness and safety of several newer monoclonal antibodies including ofatumumab [136], obinutuzumab, epratuzumab [137], and moxetumomab pasudotox [138] as single agents or in combination with a chemotherapeutic are currently under investigation. Chimeric antigen receptor (CAR) therapy has shown remarkable efficacy in B-cell ALL. CAR combines both antigen-binding and T-cell activating functions into a single receptor. CAR-modified T cells involve a mechanism in which a patient's own T cells are genetically programmed to recognize leukemic cells, inducing an antileukemic immune response. Complete remission rates as high as 90% have been reported in children and adults with relapsed and refractory ALL posttreatment with CAR-modified T cells targeting the B cell-specific antigen CD19 [139]. Treatment of the high-risk Ph-like ALL has significantly improved with the identification of genetic alterations which deregulate cytokine receptor and tyrosine kinase signaling, both common features of this subtype of ALL. Tyrosine kinase inhibitors (TKIs) such as imatinib, dasatinib, nilotinib, and ponatinib, NOTCH1 and DOT1L pathway inhibitors, and JAK inhibitors have become novel agents for Ph-like ALL therapy. In addition, 50% of Ph-like ALLs show activation of phosphatidylinositol 3-kinase/protein kinase B (PI3K/AKT) and mammalian target of rapamycin (mTOR) pathways and could therefore present potential targets for mTOR inhibitors [140]. Inhibition of the PI3K/AKT/mTOR pathways may be an effective treatment for T-ALL.

4. Protein markers of CLL and ALL as a new therapeutic targets

New specific protein markers connected with CLL and ALL which have been discovered in the last 10–15 years represent novel potential targets for highly personalized treatments of leukemia. These proteins, associated with different cellular signaling events, mostly include surface receptors/transmembrane proteins—CD5, CD19, CD20, CD22, CD23, CD52, and many others [9, 11, 31, 33, 38]—where protein phosphorylation may play an important role in protein activity regulation connected to the progression of disease and regulation of pathological events [12–14]. Focusing on such specific modifications presents key opportunities to further facilitate efficient and precise drug strategy design [55–58]. Inhibition of protein kinases associated with key phosphorylations has been an intense research topic in the last decade [67–69, 72, 73, 75]. Significant progress in protein mass spectrometry techniques, specific antibody design and development, parallel studies of genes, epigenetic proteome, and related proteins including their disease-related modifications altogether open a new horizon for a more sensitive and personalized approach to the diagnosis and treatment methods of CLL and ALL. The combination of such approaches should further facilitate the development of more efficient drugs and approaches which more specifically target the key signaling events concerning the onset and progression of the disease. Based on the fact that proteome maps are unique to each individual, there is an urgent need for personalized diagnostics and a personalized molecular treatment approach. Using the information from the proteins associated with the CLL and ALL, and the misregulation of signaling pathways in associated cell regulation events, the precise and detailed protein signaling outcome can form the base of potential success in the domain of efficient drug design and consequent molecular treatment, without the typical side effects of current conventional methods.

5. Conclusion

Given the diverse molecular and genetic alterations occurring in both CLL and ALL, it is unlikely that a single and unique therapeutic approach will be effective across all patients. Great progress has been made thus far in the identification of oncogenic drivers and therapeutic targets. However, although treatment regimens have advanced significantly, they continue to present many challenges for the majority of patients, including toxicity. Future studies focused on the identification of biomarkers should result in more effective treatments exhibiting antileukemic activity with reduced toxicity. Furthermore, highly targeted therapy can be expected to lead to improvements in remission and survival as part of individualized treatment strategies.

Conflict of interest

The authors declare no conflicts of interest.

Author details

Martina Maďarová[1], Dominik Dobransky[2] and Tomas Dobransky[1]*

1 DB Biotech Inc., Košice, Slovakia

2 BLES Biochemicals Inc., London, ON, Canada

*Address all correspondence to: tdobransky@dbbiotech.com

References

[1] Chiorazzi N, Rai KR, Ferrarini M. Chronic lymphocytic leukemia. The New England Journal of Medicine. 2005;**352**:804-815. DOI: 10.1056/NEJMra041720

[2] Damle RN, Ghiotto F, Valetto A, Albesiano E, Fais F, Yan XJ, et al. B-cell chronic lymphocytic leukemia cells express a surface membrane phenotype of activated, antigen-experienced B lymphocytes. Blood. 2002;**99**:4087-4093

[3] Seifert M, Sellmann L, Bloehdorn J, Wein F, Stilgenbauer S, Dürig J, et al. Cellular origin and pathophysiology of chronic lymphocytic leukemia. The Journal of Experimental Medicine. 2012;**209**:2183-2198. DOI: 10.1084/jem.20120833

[4] Messmer BT, Messmer D, Allen SL, Kolitz JE, Kudalkar P, Cesar D, et al. In vivo measurements document the dynamic cellular kinetics of chronic lymphocytic leukemia B cells. The Journal of Clinical Investigation. 2005;**115**:755-764. DOI: 10.1172/JCI23409

[5] Burger JA, Peled A. CXCR4 antagonists: Targeting the microenvironment in leukemia and other cancers. Leukemia. 2009;**23**:43-52. DOI: 10.1038/leu.2008.299

[6] Ten Hacken E, Burger JA. Microenvironment interactions and B-cell receptor signaling in chronic lymphocytic leukemia: Implications for disease pathogenesis and treatment. Biochimica et Biophysica Acta. 1863;**2016**:401-413. DOI: 10.1016/j.bbamcr.2015.07.009

[7] Billard C. Apoptosis inducers in chronic lymphocytic leukemia. Oncotarget. 2014;**5**:309-325. DOI: 10.18632/oncotarget.1480

[8] Burger JA, Chiorazzi N. B cell receptor signaling in chronic lymphocytic leukemia. Trends in Immunology. 2013;**34**:592-601. DOI: 10.1016/j.it.2013.07.002

[9] Stevenson FK, Krysov S, Davies AJ, Steele AJ, Packham G. B-cell receptor signaling in chronic lymphocytic leukemia. Blood. 2011;**118**:4313-4320. DOI: 10.1182/blood-2011-06-338855

[10] Hamblin TJ, Davis Z, Gardiner A, Oscier DG, Stevenson FK. Unmutated Ig V(H) genes are associated with a more aggressive form of chronic lymphocytic leukemia. Blood. 1999;**94**:1848-1854

[11] Agathangelidis A, Darzentas N, Hadzidimitriou A, Brochet X, Murray F, Yan XJ, et al. Stereotyped B-cell receptors in one-third of chronic lymphocytic leukemia: A molecular classification with implications for targeted therapies. Blood. 2012;**119**:4467-4475. DOI: 10.1182/blood-2011-11-393694

[12] Myhrvold IK, Cremaschi A, Hermansen JU, Tjønnfjord GE, Munthe LA, Taskén K, et al. Single cell profiling of phospho-protein levels in chronic lymphocytic leukemia. Oncotarget. 2018;**9**:9273-9284. DOI: 10.18632/oncotarget.23949

[13] Frank DA, Mahajan S, Ritz J. B lymphocytes from patients with chronic lymphocytic leukemia contain signal transducer and activator of transcription (STAT) 1 and STAT3 constitutively phosphorylated on serine residues. The Journal of Clinical Investigation. 1997;**100**:3140-3148. DOI: 10.1172/JCI119869

[14] Maďarová M, Mucha R, Hresko S, Makarová Z, Gdovinová Z, Szilasiová J, et al. Identification of new phosphorylation sites of CD23 in B-cells of patients with chronic lymphocytic leukemia. Leukemia

Research. 2018;**70**:25-33. DOI: 10.1016/j.leukres.2018.05.002

[15] Yamamoto JF, Goodman MT. Patterns of leukemia incidencein the United States by subtype and demographiccharacteristics, 1997-2002. Cancer Causes & Control. 2008;**19**:379-390. DOI: 10.1007/s10552-007-9097-2

[16] DeSantis CE, Lin CC, Mariotto AB, Siegel RL, Stein KD, Kramer JL, et al. Cancer treatment and survivorship statistics, 2014. CA: A Cancer Journal for Clinicians. 2014;**64**:252-271. DOI: 10.3322/caac.21235

[17] Lanasa MC. Novel insights into the biology of CLL. Hematology. American Society of Hematology. Education Program. 2010;**2010**:70-76. DOI: 10.1182/asheducation-2010.1.70

[18] Eichhorst B, Robak T, Montserrat E, Ghia P, Hillmen P, Hallek M, et al. Chronic lymphocytic leukaemia: ESMO clinical practice guidelines for diagnosis, treatment and follow-up. Annals of Oncology. 2015;**26**:v78-v84. DOI: 10.1093/annonc/mdv303

[19] Schinasi LH, De Roos AJ, Ray RM, Edlefsen KL, Parks CG, Howard BV, et al. Insecticide exposure and farm history in relation to risk of lymphomas and leukemias in the Women's health initiative observational study cohort. Annals of Epidemiology. 2015;**25**(11):803-810. DOI: 10.1016/j.annepidem. 2015.08.002

[20] Hallek M, Cheson BD, Catovsky D, Caligaris-Cappio F, Dighiero G, Dohner H, et al. International Workshop on Chronic Lymphocytic Leukemia: Guidelines for the diagnosis and treatment of chronic lymphocytic leukemia: A report fromthe international workshop on chronic lymphocyticleukemia updating the national cancer institute-workinggroup 1996 guidelines. Blood. 2008;**111**:5446-5456. DOI: 10.1182/blood-2007-06-093906

[21] Swerdlow SH, Campo E, Harris NL, Jaffe ES, Pileri SA, Stein H, et al. The 2016 revision of the World Health Organization classification of lymphoid neoplasms. Blood. 2016;**127**:2375-2390. DOI: 10.1182/blood-2016-01-643569

[22] Rai KR, Sawitsky A, Cronkite EP, Chanana AD, Levy RN, Pasternack BS. Clinical staging of chronic lymphocytic leukemia. Blood. 1975;**46**(2):219-234. DOI: 10.1182/blood-2016-08-737650

[23] Binet JL, Auquier A, Dighiero G, Chastang C, Piguet H, Goasguen J, et al. A new prognostic classification of chronic lymphocytic leukemia derived from a multivariate survival analysis. Cancer. 1981;**48**:198-206

[24] Rozman C, Montserrat E. Chronic lymphocytic leukemia. The New England Journal of Medicine. 1995;**333**(16):1052-1057. DOI: 10.1056/NEJM199510193331606

[25] Landgren O, Albitar M, Ma W, Abbasi F, Hayes RB, Ghia P, et al. B-cell clones as early markers for chronic lymphocytic leukemia. The New England Journal of Medicine. 2009;**360**:659-667. DOI: 10.1056/NEJMoa0806122

[26] Strati P, Shanafelt TD. Monoclonal B-cell lymphocytosis andearly-stage chronic lymphocytic leukemia: Diagnosis, natural history, and risk stratification. Blood. 2015;**126**:454-462. DOI: 10.1182/blood-2015-02-585059

[27] National Comprehensive Cancer Network (NCCN). NCCN Clinical Practice Guidelines in Oncology (NCCN Guidelines): Chronic Lymphocytic Leukemia/Small Lymphocytic Lymphoma. Version 2.2017. 2017. NCCN website. www.nccn.org/professionals/physician_gls/pdf/cll.pdf [Accessed May 15, 2017]

[28] Keating MJ. Chronic lymphocytic leukemia. Seminars in Oncology. 1999;**26**:107-114

[29] Hallek M, Langenmayer I, Nerl C, Knauf W, Dietzfelbinger H, Adorf D, et al. Elevated serum thymidine kinase levels identify a subgroup at high risk of disease progression in early, nonsmoldering chronic lymphocytic leukemia. Blood. 1999;**93**:1732-1737

[30] Sarfati M, Chevret S, Chastang C, Biron G, Stryckmans P, Delespesse G, et al. Prognostic importance of serum soluble CD23 level in chronic lymphocytic leukemia. Blood. 1996;**88**:4259-4264

[31] Damle RN, Wasil T, Fais F, Ghiotto F, Valetto A, Allen SL, et al. Ig V gene mutation status and CD38 expression as novel prognostic indicators in chronic lymphocytic leukemia. Blood. 1999;**94**:1840-1847

[32] Crespo M, Bosch F, Villamor N, Bellosillo B, Colomer D, Rozman M, et al. ZAP-70 expression as a surrogate for immunoglobulin-variable-region mutations in chronic lymphocytic leukemia. The New England Journal of Medicine. 2003;**348**:1764-1775

[33] Bulian P, Shanafelt TD, Fegan C, Zucchetto A, Cro L, Nückel H, et al. CD49d is the strongest flow cytometry-based predictor of overall survival in chronic lymphocytic leukemia. Journal of Clinical Oncology. 2014;**32**:897-904. DOI: 10.1200/JCO.2013.50.8515

[34] Döhner H, Stilgenbauer S, Benner A, Leupolt E, Kröber A, Bullinger L, et al. Genomic aberrations and survival in chronic lymphocytic leukemia. The New England Journal of Medicine. 2000;**343**:1910-1916. DOI: 10.1056/NEJM200012283432602

[35] Montserrat E, Rozman C. Bone marrow biopsy in chroniclymphocytic leukemia: A review of its prognosticimportance. Blood Cells. 1987;**12**:315-326

[36] Nabhan C, Rosen ST. Chronic lymphocytic leukemia: A clinical review. Journal of the American Medical Association. 2014;**312**:2265-2276. DOI: 10.1001/jama.2014.14553

[37] Rassenti LZ, Huynh L, Toy TL, Chen L, Keating MJ, Gribben JG, et al. ZAP-70 compared with immunoglobulin heavy-chain gene mutation status as a predictor of disease progression in chronic lymphocytic leukemia. The New England Journal of Medicine. 2004;**35**:893-901. DOI: 10.1056/NEJMoa040857

[38] Deaglio S, Vaisitti T, Aydin S, Bergui L, D'Arena G, Bonello L, et al. CD38 and ZAP-70 are functionally linked and mark CLL cells with high migratory potential. Blood. 2007;**110**:4012-4021. DOI: 10.1182/blood-2007-06-094029

[39] Sivina M, Hartmann E, Kipps TJ, Rassenti L, Krupnik D, Lerner S, et al. CCL3 (MIP-1alpha) plasma levels and the risk for disease progression in chronic lymphocytic leukemia. Blood. 2011;**117**:1662-1669. DOI: 10.1182/blood-2010-09-307249

[40] Yan XJ, Dozmorov I, Li W, Yancopoulos S, Sison C, Centola M, et al. Identification of outcome-correlated cytokine clusters in chronic lymphocytic leukemia. Blood. 2011;**118**:5201-5210. DOI: 10.1182/blood-2011-03-342436

[41] Fais F, Ghiotto F, Hashimoto S, Sellars B, Valetto A, Allen SL, et al. Chronic lymphocytic leukemia B cells express restricted sets of mutated and unmutated antigen receptors. The Journal of Clinical Investigation. 1998;**102**:1515-1525. DOI: 10.1172/JCI3009

[42] Binder M, Léchenne B, Ummanni R, Scharf C, Balabanov S, Trusch M, et al. Stereotypical chronic lymphocytic leukemia B-cell receptors recognize survival promoting antigens on stromal cells. PLoS One. 2010;**5**:e15992. DOI: 10.1371/journal.pone.0015992

[43] Sthoeger ZM, Wakai M, Tse DB, Vinciguerra VP, Allen SL, Budman DR, et al. Production of autoantibodies by CD5-expressing B lymphocytes from patients with chronic lymphocytic leukemia. The Journal of Experimental Medicine. 1989;**169**:255-268

[44] Chiorazzi N, Ferrarini M. B cell chronic lymphocytic leukemia: Lessons learned from studies of the B cell antigen receptor. Annual Review of Immunology. 2003;**21**:841-894. DOI: 10.1146/annurev.immunol.21.120601.141018

[45] Bröker BM, Klajman A, Youinou P, Jouquan J, Worman CP, Murphy J, et al. Chronic lymphocytic leukemic (CLL) cells secrete multispecific autoantibodies. Journal of Autoimmunity. 1988;**1**:469-481

[46] Stilgenbauer S, Lichter P, Döhner H. Genetic features of B-cell chronic lymphocytic leukemia. Reviews in Clinical and Experimental Hematology. 2000;**4**:48-72

[47] Chiorazzi N. Implications of new prognostic markers in chronic lymphocytic leukemia. Hematology. American Society of Hematology. Education Program. 2012;**2012**:76-87. DOI: 10.1182/asheducation-2012.1.76

[48] Zenz T, Krober A, Scherer K, Habe S, Buhler A, Benner A, et al. Monoallelic TP53 inactivation is associated with poorprognosis in chronic lymphocytic leukemia: Results from adetailed genetic characterization with long-term follow-up. Blood. 2008;**112**:3322-3329. DOI: 10.1182/blood-2008-04-154070

[49] Puente XS, Pinyol M, Quesada V, Conde L, Ordóñez GR, Villamor N, et al. Whole-genome sequencing identifies recurrent mutations in chronic lymphocytic leukaemia. Nature. 2011;**475**(7354):101-105. DOI: 10.1038/nature10113

[50] Quesada V, Conde L, Villamor N, Ordóñez GR, Jares P, Bassaganyas L, et al. Exome sequencing identifies recurrent mutations of the splicing factor SF3B1 gene in chronic lymphocytic leukemia. Nature Genetics. 2011;**44**:47-52. DOI: 10.1038/ng.1032

[51] Rossi D, Fangazio M, Rasi S, Vaisitti T, Monti S, Cresta S, et al. Disruption of BIRC3 associates with fludarabine chemorefractoriness in TP53 wild-type chronic lymphocytic leukemia. Blood. 2012;**119**:2854-2862. DOI: 10.1182/blood-2011-12-395673

[52] CLL Trialists' Collaborative Group. Chemotherapeuticoptions in chronic lymphocytic leukemia: A meta-analysis of the randomized trials. Journal of the National Cancer Institute. 1999;**91**(10):861-868. DOI: 10.1093/jnci/91.10.861

[53] Hallek M. Chronic lymphocytic leukemia: 2015 update ondiagnosis, risk stratification, and treatment. American Journal of Hematology. 2015;**90**(5):446-460. DOI: 10.1002/ajh.23979

[54] Eichhorst BF, Busch R, Hopfinger G, Pasold R, Hensel M, Steinbrecher C, et al. Fludarabine plus cyclophosphamideversus fludarabine alone in first-line therapy of youngerpatients with chronic lymphocytic leukemia. Blood. 2006;**107**:885-891. DOI: 10.1182/blood-2005-06-2395

[55] Tam CS, O'Brien S, Wierda W, Kantarjian H, Wen S, Do KA, et al. Long-term results of the fludarabine, cyclophosphamide, and rituximab regimen as initial therapy of chronic

lymphocytic leukemia. Blood. 2008;**112**:975-980. DOI: 10.1182/blood-2008-02-140582

[56] Hallek M, Fischer K, Fingerle-Rowson G, Fink AM, Busch R, Mayer J, et al. Addition of rituximab to fludarabine andcyclophosphamide in patients with chronic lymphocyticleukaemia: A randomised, open-label, phase 3 trial. Lancet. 2010;**376**:1164-1174. DOI: 10.1016/S0140-6736(10)61381-5

[57] Wierda WG, Kipps TJ, Mayer J, Stilgenbauer S, Williams CD, Hellmann A, et al. Ofatumumab as single-agent CD20 immunotherapy in fludarabine-refractory chronic lymphocytic leukemia. Journal of Clinical Oncology. 2010;**28**:1749-1755. DOI: 10.1200/JCO.2009.25.3187

[58] Mossner E, Brunker P, Moser S, Puntener U, Schmidt C, Herter S, et al.: Increasing the efficacy of CD20 antibodytherapy through the engineering of a new type II anti-CD20 antibody with enhanced direct and immune effector effector cell-mediated B-cell cytotoxicity. Blood. 2010;**115**:4393-4402. DOI: 10.1182/blood-2009-06-225979

[59] Osterborg A, Dyer MJ, Bunjes D, Pangalis GA, Bastion Y, Catovsky D, et al. Phase II multicenter study of human CD52 antibody in previously treated chronic lymphocytic leukemia. European study group of campath-1 h treatment in chronic lymphocytic leukemia. Journal of Clinical Oncology. 1997;**15**:1567-1574. DOI: 10.1200/JCO.1997.15.4.1567

[60] Fecteau JF, Corral LG, Ghia EM, Gaidarova S, Futalan D, Bharati IS, et al. Lenalidomide inhibits the proliferation of CLL cells via a cereblon/p21(WAF1/Cip1)-dependent mechanism independent of functional p53. Blood. 2014;**124**:1637-1644. DOI: 10.1182/blood-2014-03-559591

[61] Sher T, Miller KC, Lawrence D, Whitworth A, Hernandez-Ilizaliturri F, Czuczman MS, et al. Efficacy of lenalidomide in patients with chronic lymphocytic leukemia with high-risk cytogenetics. Leukemia & Lymphoma. 2010;**51**:85-88. DOI: 10.3109/10428190903406806

[62] Burger JA, Ghia P, Rosenwald A, Caligaris-Cappio F. The microenvironment in mature B-cell malignancies: A target for new treatment strategies. Blood. 2009;**114**:3367-3375. DOI: 10.1182/blood-2009-06-225326

[63] Stamatopoulos B, Meuleman N, De Bruyn C, Pieters K, Mineur P, Le Roy C, et al. AMD3100 disrupts the cross-talk between chronic lymphocytic leukemia cells and a mesenchymal stromal or nurse-like cell-based microenvironment: Pre-clinical evidence for its association with chronic lymphocytic leukemia treatments. Haematologica. 2012;**97**:608-615. DOI: 10.3324/haematol.2011.052779

[64] Roberts AW, Davids MS, Pagel JM, Kahl BS, Puvvada SD, Gerecitano JF, et al. Targeting BCL2 with venetoclax inrelapsed chronic lymphocytic leukemia. The New England Journal of Medicine. 2016;**374**:311-322. DOI: 10.1056/NEJMoa1513257

[65] Byrd JC, Brown JR, O'Brien S, Barrientos JC, Kay NE, Reddy NM, et al. Ibrutinib versus ofatumumab in previously treated chronic lymphoid leukemia. New England Journal of Medicine. 2014;**371**:213-223. DOI: 10.1056/NEJMoa1400376

[66] Burger JA, Keating MJ, Wierda WG, Hartmann E, Hoellenriegel J, Rosin NY, et al. Safety and activity of Ibrutinib plus rituximab for patients with high-risk chronic lymphocytic leukaemia: A single-arm, phase 2 study. Lancet Oncology. 2014;**15**:1090-1099. DOI: 10.1016/S1470-2045(14)70335-3

[67] Rushworth SA, Bowles KM, Barrera LN, Murray MY, Zaitseva L, MacEwan DJ. BTK inhibitor ibrutinib is cytotoxic to myeloma and potently enhances bortezomib and lenalidomide activities through NF-κB. Cellular Signalling. 2013;**25**:106-112. DOI: 10.1016/j.cellsig.2012.09.008

[68] Honigberg LA, Smith AM, Sirisawad M, Verner E, Loury D, Chang B, et al. The Bruton tyrosine kinase inhibitor PCI-32765 blocks B-cell activation and is efficacious in models of autoimmune disease and B-cell malignancy. Proceedings of the National Academy of Sciences of the United States of America. 2010;**107**:13075-13080. DOI: 10.1073/pnas.1004594107

[69] Ponader S, Chen SS, Buggy JJ, Balakrishnan K, Gandhi V, Wierda WG, et al. The Bruton tyrosine kinase inhibitor PCI-32765 thwarts chronic lymphocytic leukemia cell survival and tissue homing in vitro and in vivo. Blood. 2012;**119**:1182-1189. DOI: 10.1182/blood-2011-10-386417

[70] Farooqui MZ, Valdez J, Martyr S, Aue G, Saba N, Niemann CU, et al. Ibrutinib for previously untreated and relapsed or refractory chronic lymphocytic leukaemia with TP53 aberrations: A phase 2, single-arm trial. The Lancet Oncology. 2015;**16**:169-176. DOI: 10.1016/S1470-2045(14)71182-9

[71] Byrd JC, Harrington B, O'brien S, Jones JA, Schuh A, Devereux S, et al. Acalabrutinib (ACP-196) in relapsed chronic lymphocytic leukemia. The New England Journal of Medicine. 2016;**374**:323-332. DOI: 10.1056/NEJMoa1509981

[72] Lannutti BJ, Meadows SA, Herman SE, Kashishian A, Steiner B, Johnson AJ, et al. CAL-101, a p110delta selective phosphatidylinositol-3-kinase inhibitor for the treatment of B-cell malignancies, inhibits PI3K signaling and cellular viability. Blood. 2011;**117**:591-594. DOI: 10.1182/blood-2010-03-275305

[73] Hoellenriegel J, Meadows SA, Sivina M, Wierda WG, Kantarjian H, Keating MJ, et al. The phosphoinositide 3′-kinase delta inhibitor, CAL-101, inhibits B-cell receptor signaling and chemokine networks in chronic lymphocytic leukemia. Blood. 2011;**118**:3603-3612. DOI: 10.1182/blood-2011-05-352492

[74] O'Brien SM, Lamanna N, Kipps TJ, Flinn I, Zelenetz AD, Burger JA, et al. A phase 2 study of idelalisib plus rituximabin treatment-naive older patients with chronic lymphocyticleukemia. Blood. 2015;**126**:2686-2694. DOI: 10.1182/blood-2015-03-630947

[75] Balakrishnan K, Peluso M, Fu M, Rosin NY, Burger JA, Wierda WG, et al. The phosphoinositide 3 kinase (PI3K)-delta and gamma inhibitor, IPI-145 (Duvelisib), overcomes signals from the PI3K/AKT/S6 pathway and promotes apoptosis in CLL. Leukemia. 2015;**29**:1811-1822. DOI: 10.1038/leu.2015.105

[76] Kurosaki T, Hikida M. Tyrosine kinases and their substrates in B lymphocytes. Immunological Reviews. 2009;**228**:132-148. DOI: 10.1111/j.1600-065X.2008.00748.x

[77] Friedberg JW, Sharman J, Sweetenham J, Johnston PB, Vose JM, Lacasce A, et al. Inhibition of Syk with fostamatinib disodium has significant clinical activity in non-Hodgkin lymphoma and chronic lymphocytic leukemia. Blood. 2010;**115**:2578-2585. DOI: 10.1182/blood-2009-08-236471

[78] Sharman J, Hawkins M, Kolibaba K, Boxer M, Klein L, Wu M, et al. An open-label phase 2 trial of entospletinib (GS-9973), a selective spleen tyrosine kinase inhibitor, in chronic lymphocytic

leukemia. Blood. 2015;**125**:2336-2343. DOI: 10.1182/blood-2014-08-595934

[79] Alvarnas JC, Brown PA, Aoun P, Ballen KK, Barta SK, Borate U, et al. Acute lymphoblastic leukemia, version 2.2015. Journal of the National Comprehensive Cancer Network. 2015;**13**:1240-1279

[80] Terwilliger T, Abdul-Hay M. Acute lymphoblastic leukemia: A comprehensive review and 2017 update. Blood Cancer Journal. 2017;**7**:e577. DOI: 10.1038/bcj.2017.53

[81] Kato M, Manabe A. Treatment and biology of pediatric acute lymphoblastic leukemia. Pediatrics International. 2018;**60**:4-12. DOI: 10.1111/ped.13457

[82] Cancer Stat Facts: Leukemia—Acute Lymphocytic Leukemia (ALL) [Internet]. Available from: https://seer.cancer.gov/statfacts/html/alyl.html

[83] Hoelzer D, Bassan R, Dombret H, Fielding A, Ribera JM, Buske C. ESMO guidelines committee: Acute lymphoblastic leukaemia in adult patients: ESMO clinical practice guidelines for diagnosis, treatment and follow-up. Annals of Oncology. 2016;**27**:v69-v82. DOI: 10.1093/annonc/mdw025

[84] Paul S, Kantarjian H, Jabbour EJ. Adult acute lymphoblastic Leukemia. Mayo Clinic Proceedings. 2016;**91**:1645-1666. DOI: 10.1016/j.mayocp.2016.09.010

[85] Pui CH, Relling MV, Downing JR. Acute lymphoblastic leukemia. The New England Journal of Medicine. 2004;**350**(15):1535-1548. DOI: 10.1056/NEJMra023001

[86] Jabbour E, O'Brien S, Konopleva M, Kantarjian H. New insights into the pathophysiology and therapy of adult acute lymphoblastic leukemia. Cancer. 2015;**121**:2517-2528. DOI: 10.1002/cncr.29383

[87] Spector LG, Ross J, Robison LL, Bhatia S. Epidemiology and Etiology, Childhood Leukemias. 2nd ed. Cambridge University Press. pp. 48-66

[88] Sehgal S, Mujtaba S, Gupta D, Aggarwal R, Marwaha RK. High incidence of Epstein Barr virus infection in childhood acute lymphocytic leukemia: A preliminary study. Indian Journal of Pathology & Microbiology. 2010;**53**:63-67. DOI: 10.4103/0377-4929.59186

[89] Chessells J, Harrison G, Richards S, Bailey C, Hill F, Gibson B, et al. Down's syndrome and acute lymphoblastic leukaemia: Clinical features and response to treatment. Archives of Disease in Childhood. 2001;**85**:321-325

[90] Alvarnas JC, Brown PA, Aoun P, Ballen KK, Barta SK, Borate U, et al. Acute lymphoid leukemia (version 2.2015). National Comprehensive Cancer Network. 2015;**13**:1240-1279

[91] Jabbour EJ, Faderl S, Kantarjian HM. Adult acute lymphoblastic leukemia. Mayo Clinic Proceedings. 2005;**80**:1517-1527

[92] Vardiman JW, Thiele J, Arber DA, Brunning RD, Borowitz MJ, Porwit A, et al. The 2008 revision of the World Health Organization (WHO) classification of myeloid neoplasms and acute leukemia: Rationale and important changes. Blood. 2009;**114**:937-951. DOI: 10.1182/blood-2009-03-209262

[93] Coustan-Smith E, Behm FG, Sanchez J, Boyett JM, Hancock ML, Raimondi SC, et al. Immunological detection of minimal residual disease in children with acute lymphoblastic leukaemia. Lancet. 1998;**351**:550-554. DOI: 10.1016/S0140-6736(97)10295-1

[94] Janossy G, Coustan-Smith E, Campana D. The reliability of cytoplasmic CD3 and CD22 antigen expression in the immunodiagnosis of acute leukemia: A study of 500 cases. Leukemia. 1989;**3**:170-181

[95] Coustan-Smith E, Mullighan CG, Onciu M, Behm FG, Raimondi SC, Pei D, et al. Campana: Early T-cell precursor leukaemia: A subtype of very high-risk acute lymphoblastic leukaemia. The Lancet Oncology. 2009;**10**:147-156. DOI: 10.1016/S1470-2045(08)70314-0

[96] Pui CH, Crist WM, Look AT. Biology and clinical significance of cytogenetic abnormalities in childhood acute lymphoblastic leukemia. Blood. 1990;**76**:1449-1463

[97] Wetzler M, Dodge RK, Mrozek K, Carroll AJ, Tantravahi R, Block AW, et al. Prospective karyotype analysis in adult acute lymphoblastic leukemia: The cancer and leukemia group B experience. Blood. 1999;**93**:3983-3993

[98] Bruggemann M, Raff T, Flohr T, Gokbuget N, Nakao M, Droese J, et al. German Multicenter study Group for Adult Acute Lymphoblastic Leukemia: Clinical significance of minimal residual disease quantification in adult patients with standard-risk acute lymphoblastic leukemia. Blood. 2006;**107**:1116-1123. DOI: 10.1182/blood-2005-07-2708

[99] Goto H. Childhood relapsed acute lymphoblastic leukemia: Biology and recent treatment progress. Pediatrics International. 2015;**57**:1059-1066. DOI: 10.1111/ped.12837

[100] Patrick K, Wade R, Goulden N, Mitchell C, Moorman AV, Rowntree C, et al. Outcome for children and young people with early T-cell precursor acute lymphoblastic leukaemia treated on a contemporary protocol, UKALL 2003. British Journal of Haematology. 2014;**166**(3):421-424. DOI: 10.1111/bjh.1288

[101] Yoda A, Yoda Y, Chiaretti S, Bar-Natan M, Mani K, Rodig SJ, et al. Functional screening identifies CRLF2 in precursor B-cell acute lymphoblastic leukemia. Proceedings of the National Academy of Sciences of the United States of America. 2010;**107**:252-257. DOI: 10.1073/pnas.0911726107

[102] Harrison CJ, Moorman AV, Schwab C, Carroll AJ, Raetz EA, Devidas M, et al. Ponte di Legno international workshop in childhood acute lymphoblastic Leukemia. An international study of intrachromosomal amplification of chromosome 21 (iAMP21): Cytogenetic characterization and outcome. Leukemia. 2014;**28**:1015-1021. DOI: 10.1038/leu.2013.317

[103] Yasuda T, Tsuzuki S, Kawazu M, Hayakawa F, Kojima S, Ueno T, et al. Recurrent DUX4 fusions in B cell acute lymphoblastic leukemia of adolescents and young adults. Nature Genetics. 2016;**48**:569-574. DOI: 10.1038/ng.3535

[104] Stock W, La M, Sanford B, Bloomfield CD, Vardiman JW, Gaynon P, et al. Cancer and leukemia group B studies: What determines the outcomes for adolescents and young adults with acute lymphoblastic leukemia treated on cooperative group protocols? A comparison of Children's cancer group and cancer and leukemia group B studies. Blood. 2008;**112**:1646-1654. DOI: 10.1182/blood-2008-01-130237

[105] Rowe JM. Prognostic factors in adult acute lymphoblastic leukaemia. British Journal of Haematology. 2010;**150**:389-405. DOI: 10.1111/j.1365-2141.2010.08246.x

[106] Pui CH, Evans WE. Treatment of acute lymphoblastic leukemia. The

New England Journal of Medicine. 2006;**354**:166-178. DOI: 10.1056/NEJMra052603

[107] Moorman AV, Richards SM, Martineau M, Cheung KL, Robinson HM, Jalali GR, et al. Outcome heterogeneity in childhood high-hyperdiploid acute lymphoblastic leukemia. Blood. 2003;**102**:2756-2762. DOI: 10.1182/blood-2003-04-1128

[108] Kato M, Imamura T, Manabe A, Hashii Y, Koh K, Sato A, et al. Prognostic impact of gained chromosomes in high-hyperdiploid childhood acute lymphoblastic leukaemia: A collaborative retrospective study of the Tokyo Children's Cancer Study Group and Japan Association of Childhood Leukaemia Study. British Journal of Haematology. 2014;**166**:295-298. DOI: 10.1111/bjh.12836

[109] Holmfeldt L, Wei L, Diaz-Flores E, Walsh M, Zhang J, Ding L, et al. The genomic landscape of hypodiploid acute lymphoblastic leukemia. Nature Genetics. 2013;**45**:242-252. DOI: 10.1038/ng.2532

[110] Shah A, John BM, Sondhi V. Acute lymphoblastic leukemia with treatment—Naive Fanconi anemia. Indian Pediatrics. 2013;**50**:508-510

[111] Bielorai B, Fisher T, Waldman D, Lerenthal Y, Nissenkorn A, Tohami T, et al. Acute lymphoblastic leukemia in early childhood as the presenting sign of ataxia telangiectasia variant. Pediatric Hematology and Oncology. 2013;**30**:574-582. DOI: 10.3109/08880018.2013.777949

[112] Bhojwani D, Pei D, Sandlund JT, Jeha S, Ribeiro RC, Rubnitz JE, et al. ETV6-RUNX1- positive childhood acute lymphoblastic leukemia: Improved outcome with contemporary therapy. Leukemia. 2012;**26**:265-270. DOI: 10.1038/leu.2011.227

[113] Rivera GK, Raimondi SC, Hancock ML, Behm FG, Pui CH, Abromowitch M, et al. Improved outcome in childhood acute lymphoblastic leukaemia with reinforced early treatment and rotational combination chemotherapy. Lancet. 1991;**337**:61-66

[114] Schultz KR, Devidas M, Bowman WP, Aledo A, Slayton WB, Sather H, et al. Philadelphia chromosome-negative very high-risk acute lymphoblastic leukemia in children and adolescents: Results from Children's Oncology Group Study AALL0031. Leukemia. 2014;**28**:964-967. DOI: 10.1038/leu.2014.29

[115] Faderl S, Jeha S, Kantarjian HM. The biology and therapy of adult acute lymphoblastic leukemia. Cancer. 2003;**98**:1337-1354. DOI: 10.1002/cncr.11664

[116] Marks DI, Moorman AV, Chilton L, Paietta E, Enshaie A, DeWald G, et al. The clinical characteristics, therapy and outcome of 85 adults with acute lymphoblastic leukemia and t(4;11)(q21;q23)/MLL-AFF1 prospectively treated in the UKALLXII/ECOG2993 trial. Haematologica. 2013;**98**:945-952. DOI: 10.3324/haematol.2012.081877

[117] Roberts KG, Mullighan CG. Genomics in acute lymphoblastic leukaemia: Insights and treatment implications. Nature Reviews. Clinical Oncology. 2015;**12**:344-357. DOI: 10.1038/nrclinonc

[118] Roberts KG, Li Y, Payne-Turner D, Harvey RC, Yang YL, Pei D, et al. Targetable kinase-activating lesions in Ph-like acute lymphoblastic leukemia. The New England Journal of Medicine. 2014;**371**:1005-1015

[119] Roberts KG, Morin RD, Zhang J, Hirst M, Zhao Y, Su X, et al. Genetic alterations activating kinase and

cytokine receptor signaling in high-risk acute lymphoblastic leukemia. Cancer Cell. 2012;**22**:153-166. DOI: 10.1016/j.ccr.2012.06.005

[120] Iacobucci I, Mullighan CG. Genetic basis of acute lymphoblastic leukemia. Journal of Clinical Oncology. 2017;**35**:975-983. DOI: 10.1200/JCO.2016.70.7836

[121] Chiaretti S, Brugnoletti F, Tavolaro S, Bonina S, Paoloni F, Marinelli M, et al. TP53 mutations are frequent in adult acute lymphoblastic leukemia cases negative for recurrent fusion genes and correlate with poor response to induction therapy. Haematologica. 2013;**98**:e59-e61. DOI: 10.3324/haematol.2012.076786

[122] Zhang J, McCastlain K, Yoshihara H, Xu B, Chang Y, Churchman ML, et al. Deregulation of DUX4 and ERG in acute lymphoblastic leukemia. Nature Genetics. 2016;**8**: 1481-1489. DOI: 10.1038/ng.3691

[123] Liu Y, Wang BY, Zhang WN, Huang JY, Li BS, Zhang M, et al. Genomic profiling of adult and pediatric B cell acute lymphoblastic leukemia. eBioMedicine. 2016;**8**:173-183. DOI: 10.1016/j.cbiom

[124] Weng AP, Ferrando AA, Lee W, Morris JPT, Silverman LB, Sanchez-Irizarry C, et al. Activating mutations of NOTCH1 in human T cell acute lymphoblastic leukemia. Science. 2004;**306**:269-271. DOI: 10.1126/science.1102160

[125] Belver L, Ferrando A. The genetics and mechanisms of T cell acute lymphoblastic leukaemia. Nature Reviews. Cancer. 2016;**16**:494-507. DOI: 10.1038/nrc.2016.63

[126] Zhang J, Ding L, Holmfeldt L, Wu G, Heatley SL, Payne-Turner D, et al. The genetic basis of early T-cell precursor acute lymphoblastic leukaemia. Nature. 2012;**481**:157-163. DOI: 10.1038/nature10725

[127] Ferrando AA, Neuberg DS, Staunton J, Loh ML, Huard C, Raimondi SC, et al. Gene expression signatures define novel oncogenic pathways in T cell acute lymphoblastic leukemia. Cancer Cell. 2002;**1**:75-87

[128] O'Connor D, Bate J, Wade R, Clack R, Dhir S, Hough R, et al. Infection-related mortality in children with acute lymphoblastic leukemia: A retrospective analysis of infectious deaths on UKALL 2003. Blood. 2014;**124**:1056-1061. DOI: 10.1038/leu.2014.29

[129] Pui CH, Nichols KE, Yang JJ. Somatic and germline genomics in paediatric acute lymphoblastic leukaemia. Nature Reviews. Clinical Oncology. 2018;**16**:227-240. DOI: 10.1038/s41571-018-0136-6

[130] Gaynon PS, Angiolillo AL, Carroll WL, Nachman JB, Trigg ME, Sather HN, et al. Long-term results of the Children's CancerGroup studies for childhood acute lymphoblastic leukemia 1983-2002: A Children's oncology group report. Leukemia. 2010;**24**(2):285-297. DOI: 10.1038/leu.2009.262

[131] Narayanan S, Shami PJ. Treatment of acute lymphoblastic leukemia in adults. Critical Reviews in Oncology/Hematology. 2012;**81**:94-102. DOI: 10.1016/j.critrevonc.2011.01.014

[132] Pui CH, Campana D, Pei D, Bowman WP, Sandlund JT, Kaste SC, et al. Treating childhood acute lymphoblastic leukemia without cranial irradiation. The New England Journal of Medicine. 2009;**360**:2730-2741. DOI: 10.1056/NEJMoa0900386

[133] Maury S, Chevret S, Thomas X, Heim D, Leguay T, Huguet F, et al. Rituximab in B-lineage adult acute lymphoblastic leukemia. The New

England Journal of Medicine. 2016;**375**(11):1044-1053. DOI: 10.1056/NEJMoa1605085

[134] Kantarjian HM, DeAngelo DJ, Stelljes M, Martinelli G, Liedtke M, Stock W, et al. Inotuzumab ozogamicin versus standard therapy for acute lymphoblastic leukemia. The New England Journal of Medicine. 2016;**375**(8):740-753. DOI: 10.1056/NEJMoa1509277

[135] Nagorsen D, Kufer P, Baeuerle PA, Bargou R. Blinatumomab: A historical perspective. Pharmacology & Therapeutics. 2012;**136**:334-342. DOI: 10.1016/j.pharmthera.2012.07.013

[136] Jabbour E, Kantarjian H, Thomas D, Sasaki K, Garcia-Manero G, Garris R, et al. Phase II study of the hyper-CVAD regimen in combination with ofatumumab as front line therapy for adults with CD-20 positive acute lymphoblastic leukemia (ALL). Blood. 2014;**124**(21):5277

[137] Raetz EA, Cairo MS, Borowitz MJ, Blaney SM, Krailo MD, Leil TA, et al. Chemoimmunotherapy reinduction with epratuzumab in children with acute lymphoblastic leukemia in marrow relapse: A Children's oncology group pilot study. Blood. 2008;**6**:3756-3762. DOI: 10.1200/JCO.2007.15.3528

[138] Wayne AS, Kreitman RJ, Findley HW, Lew G, Delbrook C, Steinberg SM, et al. Anti-CD22 immunotoxin RFB4(dsFv)-PE38 (BL22) for CD22-positive hematologic malignancies of childhood: Preclinical studies and phase I clinical trial. Clinical Cancer Research. 2010;**16**(6):1894-1903. DOI: 10.1158/1078-0432.CCR-09-2980

[139] Park JH, Geyer MB, Brentjens RJ. CD19-targeted CART-cell therapeutics for hematologic malignancies: Interpreting clinical outcomes to date. Blood. 2016;**127**(26):3312-3320. DOI: 10.1182/blood-2016-02-629063

[140] Ofran Y, Izraeli S. BCR-ABL (Ph)-like acute leukemia—Pathogenesis, diagnosis and therapeutic options. Blood Reviews. 2016;**31**:11-16. DOI: 10.1016/j.blre.2016.09.001

Chapter 6

Chronic Lymphocytic Leukemia: Rapidly Changing Treatment Landscape

Yazan Samhouri, Rupin Shah and Cyrus Khan

Abstract

Chronic lymphocytic leukemia (CLL) is the most common type of leukemia in developed countries. CLL is diagnosed with absolute B lymphocyte count (B-ALC) >5000/micrL sustained for at least 3 months, morphologically mature-appearing small lymphocytes, and flow cytometry showing the typical immunophenotype of CLL cells. Different prognostic parameters are used to differentiate between low-and high-risk patients, which would affect treatment decisions. Rai and Binet staging systems are the two most commonly used in practice. There has been a significant change in how we manage patients in CLL over the last 5 years. We have shifted away from chemoimmunotherapy toward novel agents such as BTK, PIK3, and BCL-2 inhibitors, which are not only more efficacious but are also safer and better tolerated. New prognostic models are being developed, and it appears that minima residual disease (MRD) directed therapy will become the norm in the future. Many clinical trials are looking at various combinations of novel therapies, with a defined period of treatment based on MRD analysis, to enable patients to have a period of treatment-free remission instead of continuous therapy. In this chapter, we summarize the latest updates in CLL management.

Keywords: CLL, leukemia, treatment, chemoimmunotherapy, MRD, novel agents

1. Introduction

With an age-adjusted incidence of 4–5 per 100,000 population, chronic lymphocytic leukemia (CLL) is the most common type of leukemia in developed countries. The median age at diagnosis is 72 years, and more men than women (2:1) are affected [1]. CLL is one of the B-cell chronic lymphoproliferative disorders. It is characterized by a progressive accumulation of functionally incompetent lymphocytes, which are usually monoclonal in origin.

2. Diagnosis

CLL diagnosis depends on the presentation. For patients presenting with absolute lymphocytosis; CBC, flow cytometry of the peripheral blood, and examination of the peripheral smear are adequate to diagnose CLL [2]. Diagnosis of CLL using these tests requires identification of absolute B lymphocyte count (B-ALC) >5000/micrL sustained for at least 3 months, morphologically mature-appearing

 IntechOpen

small lymphocytes, and flow cytometry showing the typical immunophenotype of CLL cells: extremely low levels of surface membrane immunoglobulin (SmIg) and either Kappa or Lambda (but not both), CD19, CD20, CD23 and CD5 positive cells. Evaluation of the bone marrow is not usually necessary, but is included in the evaluation of patients with unexplained cytopenias. Patients presenting with lymphadenopathy without lymphocytosis will need ideally an excisional lymph node biopsy or alternatively a needle biopsy showing mature lymphocytes with the previously mentioned phenotype to diagnose small lymphocytic lymphoma (SLL) which is considered by WHO the same disease as CLL with different manifestations [3].

Monoclonal B cell lymphocytosis is diagnosed when B-ALC is <5000/micrL persistently with no other manifestations of disease activity such as lymphadenopathy, hepatosplenomegaly, disease related cytopenias, or disease related symptoms. Patients with disease related cytopenias are diagnosed with CLL regardless of B-ALC and patients with any of the other manifestations are considered to have SLL [2]. Before 2008, the diagnosis of CLL was based on ALC equal or more than 5000/microL in the setting of appropriate immunophenotype. Patients with an absolute B lymphocyte count (B-ALC) less than 5000/microL and an ALC more than 5000/microL represented an overlap between CLL and monoclonal B cell lymphocytosis. The switch to using B-ALC for the diagnosis of CLL in 2008 eliminated this overlap [4, 5].

3. Prognostication

CLL is commonly thought of as an indolent disease associated with a prolonged clinical course and that patients with CLL will die from unrelated cause rather than the disease itself. It is important to know that this only happens in one third of the patients. More commonly, patients will have two phases of the disease: an initial asymptomatic phase (5–10 years) where the course will be benign, followed by the terminal phase (1–2 years) where performance status will decline due to recurring need for hospitalization. Some patients die quickly within 1–2 years of the diagnosis. Because of this variable natural clinical course of CLL, there have been always efforts to come up with reliable and clinically applicable criteria that would allow recognizing those patients with poor prognosis to start treatment as soon as possible and improve their survival and differentiate them from the other group where the prognosis is good and treatment can be delayed to avoid treatment toxicity [6–8].

3.1 Rai and Binet staging systems

Rai and Binet staging systems are the most commonly used systems in practice and the international workshop Group on CLL (iwCLL) recommends using an integrated system using both methods [9]. Both systems depend on findings of CBC and physical exam findings only, addition of CT scan of the chest, abdomen, and pelvis is not routinely recommended to stratify patients.

Rai staging system divides patients into 5 groups (**Table 1**). It was published initially in 1975, with initial reports showing one quarter of patients fall in stage 0 on presentation, half of patients fall in stages 1 and 2, and a quarter of them fall in stages 3 and 4. Later reports showed that more patients fall in earlier stages because of earlier diagnosis due to the more routine testing being done in recent years including CBC [10]. Median survival decreases from almost 12 years in stage 0 to a year and a half in stages 3 and 4 [11]. In 1980s, this staging system was modified to include three stages based on actuarial survival pattern: Low risk (Rai stage 0), intermediate risk (Rai stages 1 and 2), and high risk (Rai stage 3 and 4). Of note,

Stage	Clinical features	Median survival (in years)
0 (low risk)	Lymphocytosis only	>10
I and II (intermediate risk)	Lymphadenopathy (I) and hepatosplenomegaly (II)	5–8
III and IV (high risk)	Anemia (III), thrombocytopenia (IV)	1.5

Table 1.
Rai staging system.

Stage	Clinical features	Median survival (in years)
A	<3 areas of lymphadenopathy; no anemia or thrombocytopenia	Comparable to age-matched controls
B	Three or more areas of lymphadenopathy; no anemia or thrombocytopenia	7
C	Hemoglobin <100 g/L or platelets <100 x 10^9 g/L	2

Table 2.
Binet staging system.

if complete or partial remission is achieved with successful therapy, and a patient's stage shifts from a higher risk to a lower risk category, the outlook for survival improves accordingly [12].

Binet staging system takes into consideration five potential sites of involvement: cervical, axillary, and inguinal lymphadenopathy (each area counts as one either unilateral or bilateral), spleen, and liver, in addition to the presence of anemia and/or thrombocytopenia. Based on these factors, Binet staging system divide patients into three groups (**Table 2**) [13].

One important practical concept is to reliably differentiate between autoimmune cytopenias and cytopenias related to CLL because patients with autoimmune cytopenias have better outcome than Binet stage C patients although still worse than stage A and they can normalize their counts with treatments directed at the autoimmune cytopenia thus delay CLL treatment [14, 15].

Both systems are not very effective for predicting early disease progression. Although routine imaging is not recommended for staging of patients with CLL, visceral adenopathy may occur in early-stage disease and might predict an early disease progression. It is not known if the presence of visceral adenopathy warrants any specific change in therapy [16].

3.2 Other prognostic factors

Historically, the presence of CD38 by flow cytometry appeared to be independently associated with an adverse prognosis as well as Increased levels of ZAP-70 detected by flow cytometry [17]. It is a tyrosine kinase normally expressed by NK and T cells, and required for normal T cell receptor signaling. ZAP-70 is not normally expressed in B lymphocytes, but has been found in a subset of patients with CLL. The clinical significance of CD38 and ZAP-70 have declined overtime with better understanding of CLL cytogenetics.

Currently, we use cytogenetics, molecular studies, lymphocyte doubling time, and beta-2 microglobulin [18]. Patients with del(13q) have favorable outcome, patients with trisomy 12 have intermediate outcome while patients with del(11q) and del(17p)/P53 have poor outcome. The prognosis of patients with del(11q) has improved with the use of certain treatment regimens (e.g., fludarabine, cyclophosphamide, rituximab) while that of del(17p) or TP53 mutations remains poor despite such treatments. Analysis of CLL8 trial showed worse outcome in patients with SF3B1 and RPS15 gene mutations. Also, patients with complex karyotype and NOTCH1 mutations have more aggressive course.

The lymphocyte doubling time is the number of months it takes the absolute lymphocyte count to double. Doubling time <12 months is associated with a progressive course and a longer doubling time is associated with an indolent course. This factor is somewhat limited in usefulness because it takes time to measure. In patients with early stage disease, the presence of a short doubling time may favor more aggressive therapy. Higher levels of Beta-2 microglobulin (B2M) are associated with poorer outcome. B2M should be interpreted with caution in the context of renal disease, or alternatively GFR-adjusted B2M can be used although lacks validation in prospective studies [19]. Moreover, approximately half of CLL clones will demonstrate unmutated immunoglobulin heavy chain variable regions (IGHV), a finding associated with shorter survival overall and a higher risk of relapse following conventional treatment, including chemoimmunotherapy and hematopoietic cell transplantation [20].

3.3 International prognostic index for chronic lymphocytic leukemia (CLL-IPI)

An international group of investigators did a comprehensive analysis [21] to develop a prognostic index for CLL. Using data from 3472 treatment naive patients participating in prospective, randomized clinical trials, five independent prognostic factors were identified: TP53 deletion or mutation, or both, IGHV mutational status, serum B2M concentration, clinical stage, and age. Using weighted grading of the independent factors, a prognostic index was derived that separated patients into four risk groups with significantly different overall survival at 5 years: low (93%), intermediate (79%), high (63%), and very high risk (23%). This chronic lymphocytic leukemia international prognostic index (CLL-IPI) has now been validated by several other groups and is expected to improve patient counseling and the planning of clinical trials. Other risk scores have been proposed, but none of them has been generally accepted. Of note, none of the scores (including the CLL-IPI) affects the decision of when to initiate therapy.

4. CLL therapy

4.1 Early evolution

In the 1940's, steroids were the first systemic therapy for CLL. The risk of infection, other adverse effects from long term steroid use as well as transient nature of responses, steroids do not have a central role in the treatment of CLL. They can be used along with anti-CD 20 Ab to achieve remission in some patients.

Steroids were followed by the use of alkylating agent chlorambucil in the treatment of CLL, either in combination or as a single agent. These treatments produced objective response rates but mostly resulted on partial responses [22, 23]. This was followed by a long time period before newer drugs were introduced in the treatment of CLL. Fludarabine has been used in various combinations to improve outcomes in CLL. When compared to CAP (cyclophosphamide, doxorubicin and prednisone), fludarabine showed favorable results [24]. Even when it was compared to chlorambucil, fludarabine induced higher response rates but did not offer any survival advantage at the expense of higher toxicities especially from infection and neutropenia [25]. Cladribine in combination with prednisone achieved response rates similar to fludarabine when compared to chlorambucil but failed to demonstrate any survival benefit [26, 27]. Cyclophosphamide combined with fludarabine in previously untreated patients showed lower prevalence of residual disease and increased progression free survival (PFS) but again no benefit in overall survival (OS) [28]. When rituximab was combined with fludarabine and cyclophosphamide there was an improvement in PFS as well as OS [29]. This was observed across multiple phase 3 randomized trials [30, 31]. Subset analysis of these trials led to the discovery that patients with mutated IGHV status, FCR led to long term remissions [30, 32].

4.2 Upfront treatment

Indication for treatment of CLL include severe fatigue, weight loss, night sweats, fever without infection, threatened organ function, progressive lymphadenopathy, anemia or thrombocytopenia that is progressive in nature, autoimmune anemia or thrombocytopenia not responsive to steroids [2]. In addition to these factors, patient age, performance status, presence or absence of del(17p) or TP53 mutation, IGHV mutation status should be assessed prior to initiating treatment in patients with indications to treat. Imaging should be considered as well to evaluate disease burden.

4.2.1 CLL without del(17p) or TP53 mutation

The CLL 8 trial was a pivotal one that established chemoimmunotherapy as the standard of care for patients that can tolerate it. The FCR regimen (fludarabine, cyclophosphamide and rituxan) was compared against FC (fludarabine, cyclophosphamide). Previously untreated CLL patients were randomized to either receive 6 cycles of FCR or FC. The FCR regimen resulted in higher ORR (90% v/s 80%) and CR rates 94% v/s 22%). The median OS was not reached for FCR and was about 86 months for the FC regimen. Subset analysis showed that the maximal benefit was derived by fit patients with CLL, especially those with mutated IGHV [32]. The FCR regimen however has its share of side effects and cannot be given to older patients.

The CCL2M trial looked at the feasibility of Bendamustine-Rituxan (BR) in untreated CLL patients and the results were found to be encouraging [33]. This prompted its comparison to other treatment regimens. The MABLE study looked at BR versus Chlorambucil-Rituxan in patients ineligible to receive fludarabine. Complete response rates were higher in the BR arm (24%) as compared to the chlorambucil-rituxan arm. Overall response rate and overall survival were not different among the two arms. However the PFS (40 months v/s 30 months) and Minimal Residual Disease (MRD) negativity (66% v/s 36%) were higher in the BR arm as compared to the Chlorambucil- rituxan arm [34].

CLL10 trial compared BR with FCR. The primary end point was PFS with the objective to assess non inferiority of BR as compared to FCR. The trial confirmed the superiority of FCR therapy (Median PFS 55 vs. 42 months) in fit patients and in patients with IGHV mutated status. However, in patients over 65 years of age the toxicity profile was better with BR.

The CLL11 trial found that chlorambucil-obinutuzumab had better PFS (26.7 months) as compared to rituximab-chlorambucil (16.3 months). The PFS for chlorambucil monotherapy was the shortest (11.1 months). The obinutuzumab-chlorambucil arm also had trend towards OS benefit as compared to the other 2 arms. The study population included CLL patients with comorbidities [35]. Based on these 2 trials both BR and chlorambucil- rituxan or obinutuzumab-chlorambucil are acceptable alternatives in elderly patients or those with comorbidities.

On a similar note, the COMPLEMENT 1 trial showed the combining ofatumumab to chlorambucil in fludarabine ineligible patients showed better PFS (22.4 months) as compared to the monotherapy arm (13.1 months) [36].

However, with the advent of novel agents the landscape of treatment in CLL has significantly changed. The RESONATE-2 study compared single agent chlorambucil to ibrutinib which is a Bruton's Tyrosine Kinase inhibitor. The ORR (92% v/s 36%) as well as PFS at 2 years (89% v/s 34%) in favor of ibrutinib (**Figure 1**). Based on the results of this study ibrutinib was approved for use in the first line setting of CLL. Results from the ECOG ACRIN Cancer research group trial E1912 were recently published. The study compared FCR versus Ibrutinib + Rituxan (IR) in treatment naive patients without deletion 17p. IR was found to be superior to FCR in all subgroups except for the IGHV mutated group. IR group saw significant less neutropenia and infectious complications as well as compared to FCR [38].

The alliance intergroup study showed that in older patients above 65, ibrutinib should be the standard of care as PFS was better in the ibrutinib arms then the BR arms [39]. However this study did not suggest a benefit of adding anti-CD 20 MAB therapy to ibrutinib monotherapy. In the older patient group, where chlorambucil is a treatment option, the iLLUMINATE trial showed that ibrutinib plus obinutuzumab combination resulted in better PFS as compared to chlorambucil plus obinutuzumab, albeit with greater serious adverse events [40]. Between the RESONATE-2 study and ECOG ACRIN study, ibrutinib has been established a first line recommendation in both younger as well as older patients with CLL.

Recently, CLL14 trial studied the combination of fixed-duration venetoclax and obinutuzumab versus obinutuzumab and chlorambucil in 432 treatment-naïve patients with CLL and coexisting medical conditions. Patients were evenly randomized to receive 12 months of venetoclax alongside 6 months of obinutuzumab or 6 months of obinutuzumab followed by 6 months of chlorambucil. Results from the trial showed the venetoclax combination reduced the risk of disease progression or death by 67% versus obinutuzumab plus chlorambucil in patients with treatment-naïve CLL and co-existing medical conditions (HR, 0.33; 95% CI, 0.22-0.51; P < .0001). The overall response rate (ORR) was 85% with venetoclax/obinutuzumab versus 71% in the control arm (P = .0007). The complete response (CR) or CR with incomplete hematologic recovery (CRi) rates were 50% versus 23%, respectively. The rate of minimal residual disease (MRD)-negativity in the bone marrow was 57% in the venetoclax arm compared with 17% in the obinutuzumab/chlorambucil arm. The MRD-negativity rates in the peripheral blood were

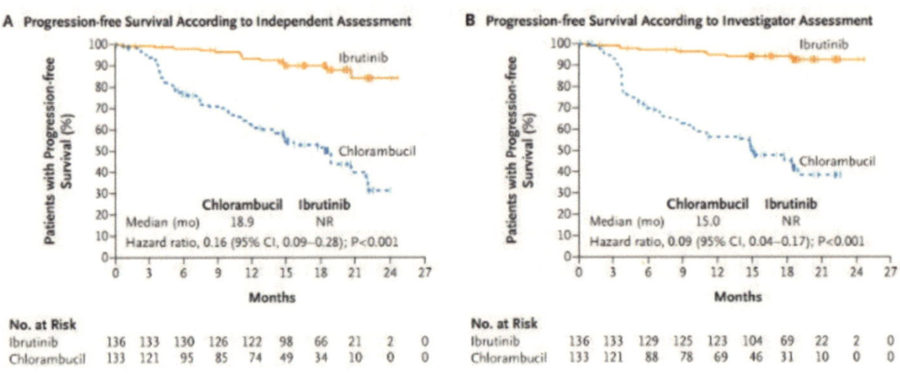

Figure 1.
Progression-free survival of Ibrutinib vs. Chlorambucil [37].

76% versus 35%, respectively. Venetoclax and obinutuzumab combination is the only chemotherapy-free option with fixed duration that proven to provide such a durable response.

4.2.2 CLL with del(17p) or TP53 mutation

Ibrutinib provides durable responses and is well tolerated in patients with del(17p). Historically this group of patients generally have poorer outcomes as compared to patients with CLL but without del(17p) [41]. Other treatments in the front-line setting are listed in NCCN for these patients however none of them are very effective. The CAPTIVATE trial is currently on going looking at venetoclax along with ibrutinib in the upfront setting.

Is summary, as far as front line therapy is concerned, for fit patients with IGVH mutated status it is reasonable to use chemo-immunotherapy such as FCR or BR. All other patients including young or older patients with high risk disease such as those with unmutated IGHD, 17p del or p53 mutation or 11q deletion it's recommended to treat with a novel agent such as ibrutinib as there has been accumulating evidence of better efficacy when compared to chemoimmunotherapy alone.

4.3 Relapsed or refractory chronic lymphocytic leukemia

4.3.1 Definitions

The International Workshop on CLL (iwCLL) defines relapsed disease when it occurs in patients who have previously achieved either a complete or partial remission but then develop progressive disease after a period of 6 months or more. Patients who fail to achieve either a partial or complete remission with therapy or those who develop disease progression within 6 months of last therapy are defined to have refractory disease. This distinction is principally made because many patients with progressive disease occurring later after the discontinuation of treatment can be successfully retreated using the same medication, or by switching to other available treatments. In contrast, patients who have refractory disease are unlikely to respond to a trial of the previously used therapy and have a much poorer prognosis [2]. Of note, The iwCLL response criteria were originally developed using data from patients treated with single agents (i.e., fludarabine, chlorambucil). As first-line therapy has evolved, the overall response rate and median progression-free survival have increased. The definitions of relapsed and refractory disease will likely change as therapy improves especially that we depend on expected progression free survival (PFS) in practice more than the 6 months rule to choose the next regimen as illustrated below.

The choice of treatment at relapse should consider how soon the relapse happens after initial treatment. If it happens sooner than the expected median PFS for the specific regimen is considered "Early relapse", while it is considered "Late relapse" when it happens after the expected median PFS [42]. Prospective trials have reported median PFS for different regimens, as a rule of thumb, progression within 2–3 years of initial treatment with fludarabine, cyclophosphamide, and rituximab (FCR) or within 1 year of other chemoimmunotherapy regimens may be considered to have early relapse.

4.3.2 Targeted therapies of relapsing or refractory CLL

For early relapsing CLL, it's recommended to start a targeted therapy with either ibrutinib, idelalisib plus rituximab, or venetoclax with or without rituximab rather than retreatment with the prior therapy or a trial of another chemoimmunotherapy regimen. One series reported the median survival of 42 patients unresponsive to fludarabine as 48 weeks and only 11% responded to other chemoimmunotherapies [43]. The optimal length of treatment has not been defined but common practice to continue until disease progression or unacceptable toxicity.

Ibrutinib: it is a common treatment of choice for patients with refractory or early relapsing disease. Ibrutinib is a Bruton's tyrosine kinase (BTK) inhibitor [44]. The RESONATE trial which is a multicenter open label phase III trial showed better overall response rate (ORR), PFS, and overall survival (OS) compared to ofatumumab (an anti-CD20 monoclonal antibody) in patients with refractory/relapsed CLL, these benefits were found across all subgroups of patients, including those with high-risk features such as del(17p). This late observation was confirmed in the RENONATE-17 trial in 2016 where ORR was 83% at a median follow up of 28 months in 144 patients with relapsed/refractory CLL/SLL with del(17p) [45, 46]. Expected side effects from ibrutinib include diarrhea, fever, and nausea. Higher rates of atrial fibrillation (6–16%) and pneumonitis were noted in the clinical trials [47], atrial fibrillation is usually manageable without discontinuation of the drug. Another important side effect is increased risk of bleeding, ibrutinib should be used with caution if patient is on one anti-platelet medicine and should be avoided if on two anti-platelets or anticoagulants as fatal cases of bleeding happened in those scenarios. Also, Ibrutinib should be discontinued 3–7 days before and after surgery to decrease risk of perioperative bleeding. Patients should be also reminded to avoid NSAIDs [48]. Ibrutinib is associated with a usually "transient" lymphocytosis that peaks after approximately 4–8 weeks and resolves in the majority despite continued drug exposure with a median duration of 14 weeks. The starting dose of ibrutinib is 420 mg orally once daily, except for patients with mild liver impairment (child-pugh class A), the starting dose is reduced to 140 mg daily since it's metabolized in the liver and is contraindicated in moderate to severe liver impairment.

Idelalisib: It is an oral inhibitor of phosphoinositide 3′-kinase (PI3K) delta. It is given in combination with Rituximab. A phase 3 multicenter trial compared Idelalisib and rituximab vs. placebo and rituximab in 220 patients with relapsed CLL showed superior ORR, PFS, and OS (81%, 93%, and 92%, respectively), these benefits were seen in all prespecified subgroups, including those with 17p deletion, TP53 mutation, and IGHV mutations [49]. Possible side effects include: pneumonia and febrile neutropenia most commonly, but also fatigue, nausea, and diarrhea have been reported. Idelalisib can cause severe elevations in AST and ALT, it is reversible on holding the drug and never led to permanent discontinuation in clinical trials. The starting dose is 150 mg twice daily. Other possible combinations are Idelalisib plus Bendamustine plus Rituxan or idelalisib plus ofatumumab, those combinations led to more grade 3 toxicities and treatment related deaths, respectively, so extreme caution should be paid while choosing patients for these combinations [50, 51]. As with ibrutinib, idelalisib can cause transient lymphocytosis that peaks in the second week of treatment and resolves spontaneously by week 12, adding Rituximab decrease its severity and shortens its duration. CMV monitoring and prophylaxis against Pneumocystis pneumonia (PCP) are important with idelalisib use. It carries a boxed warning regarding hepatotoxicity, colitis, and pneumonitis.

Duvelisib: it is an oral inhibitor of PI3K delta and gamma isoforms. The phase 3 DUO trial was the largest trial to study the efficacy of duvelisib, it included 319 patients assigned to duvelisib vs. ofatumumab. Duvelisib had higher ORR and median PFS (74% and 13.3 months, respectively) [52]. Duvelisib is usually reserved for patients with multiply relapsed disease, usually after treatment with ibrutinib and venetoclax, with or without prior chemoimmunotherapy. The starting dose is 25 mg administered orally twice a day over a 28-day treatment cycle. Toxicities include opportunistic infections, diarrhea or colitis, cutaneous reactions, and pneumonitis. Hepatic function and blood counts must be monitored for hepatotoxicity and neutropenia. Like idelalisib, it is recommended to use PCP and CMV prophylaxis.

Venetoclax: it is an oral inhibitor of BCL2, an antiapoptotic protein that is pathologically overexpressed and that is central to the survival of CLL cells. Initial phase 2 trials showed ORR more than 65% for venetoclax [53, 54]. The MURANO trial, an international phase 3 trial, compared Venetoclax plus rituximab vs. bendamustine plus rituximab in 389 patients with relapsed/refractory CLL showed higher PFS of 85% and OS of 92% at 2 years for the venetoclax arm, this effect was maintained in high risk patients and older adults. Patients assigned to venetoclax arm were also more likely to achieve undetectable minimal residual disease (uMRD) which is a status predictive of superior PFS [55]. The most common toxicities are pancytopenia, diarrhea, and upper respiratory tract infection. Because venetoclax increases risk of TLS, high risk patients (i.e. any lymph node >10 cm or lymph node >5 cm and ALC >25 x 109/L) should receive the first few doses in the inpatient setting with IV hydration, use of allopurinol or rasburicase, and frequent monitoring of TLS labs. Venetoclax is started at 20 mg daily and increased gradually over 5 weeks to a final daily dose of 400 mg. Rituximab is started after the patient has completed the escalation schedule and received the 400 mg dose for 7 days. It is common practice to use venetoclax after ibrutinib failure.

4.3.3 Late relapse: Retreatment versus targeted therapy

Although both options are valid in late relapsed CLL patients, each option has its advantages and disadvantages. Targeted therapy is generally the preferred option because they have better PFS and may improve OS, the best example on that is the MURANO trial mentioned above, patients who relapsed after 24 months of initial treatment with bendamustine and rituximab were included in the study, and still they had better PFS and OS [55]. Targeted therapy also offers the convenience of an oral regimen. On the other hand, retreatment with initial chemoimmunotherapy regimen may be considered for patients who experienced minimal toxicity with the initial treatment, targeted therapy is associated with unique toxicities and is often administered without breaks until the time of progression. In a phase 2 study, patients who were initially treated with FCR and relapsed after 3 years showed median survival of 5 years and estimated five-year survival rate of 70% when they were retreated with FCR, although the toxicities, especially myelosuppression, were more frequent [56].

Fludarabine-based therapy: Fludarabine, cyclophosphamide, plus rituximab (FCR) is a preferred treatment option for younger patients (<70 years) with standard-risk CLL. Patients with del(17p) or *TP53* mutations have particularly poor outcomes following fludarabine-based therapy and should be considered for targeted therapy.

Bendamustine-based therapy: Bendamustine plus rituximab (BR) is an acceptable alternative to fludarabine-based regimens among patients with decreased renal function or other comorbidities. BR is well tolerated, but appears to be slightly less effective than fludarabine-based regimens [57]. The most common toxicities are neutropenia, thrombocytopenia, and anemia [58]. Infusion is associated with a hypersensitivity reaction in approximately 5% of patients.

Ofatumumab-based therapy: Single agent ofatumumab has demonstrated partial response rates of approximately 50% in patients with relapsed or refractory CLL, although response duration is usually short [59]. The combination of ofatumumab plus chlorambucil is expected to result in higher response rates.

Patients with CLL experience serial relapses and many will be treated with each of these agents at some point during their disease course. A preferred order for their use has not been established. A choice is primarily made based on the patient's prior treatment and the regimens' expected toxicities.

5. Role of transplant in CLL

In the setting of approval of novel agents in the treatment of CLL the number of transplants that are being performed in Europe and the United States are decreasing. In the chemoimmunotherapy era, patients with TP53 deletion/mutation, fludarabine refractoriness, early relapse (<24 months) after FCR treatment were in the highest risk group. Allogeneic Stem Cell Transplant (SCT) would be considered in these patients as the only viable treatment option. Today however, these patients have ibrutinib, idelalisib and venetoclax and various combination of novel agents with immunotherapy as possible treatment options. There are no randomized clinical trials that compare the outcomes of allogeneic SCT with conventional chemotherapy, chemoimmunotherapy or novel therapy regimens. Most transplants offered for CLL use reduced intensity conditioning (RIC), however no trials have been conducted to compare it to myeloablative conditioning. RIC resulted in reduced toxicity without compromising engraftment and anti-tumor activity [60]. Follow up results for studies with RIC indicate that about 40% of patients achieve long term disease control and RIC also overcomes the negative prognostic effect of TP53, fludarabine refractoriness as well as that of SF3B1 and NOTCH gene mutations [61–63]. Generally, allogeneic transplants are no longer offered to patients with del(17p) in first remission. In the relapsed setting the role of SCT must be weighed against the comorbidities, prior therapies, and duration of response to prior therapies as well as current mutation status including TP53, NOTCH1 and SF3B1. Patient must be informed about the side effect profile and non-relapse mortality associated with allogeneic transplant compared to the toxicity and side effect profile of novel agents. (**Figure 2**).

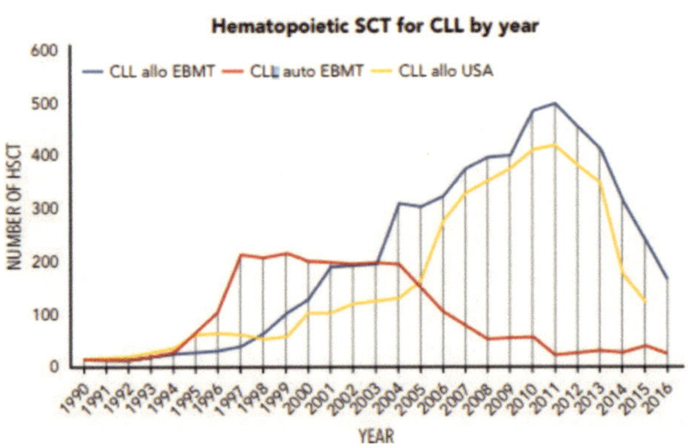

Figure 2.
Hematopoietic SCT for CLL by year [64, 65].

6. Role of minimal residual disease (MRD) testing in CLL

MRD in CLL is assessed most commonly using multiparametric flow cytometry with a sensitivity to detect <1 CLL cell in 10,000 leukocytes. MRD – undetectable (MRD-U) has been defined detection of <1 CLL cell per 10,000 leukocytes [2].

MRD-U in the blood or bone marrow strongly correlates with longer PFS in the patients treated with chemoimmunotherapy has been noted in numerous studies [30, 57, 64]. However, MRD- U is rarely achieved in patients who are on ibrutinib, a drug that offers significant clinical benefit in PFS and survival in CLL patients [66]. So, there is consensus that while MRD- U is generally a favorable outcome for patients but its exact use case scenario in clinical practice is yet to be determined. As of now the potential use of MRD status in CLL patients is in the context of clinical trials, as a surrogate for PFS depending on the type of treatment used and possibly as a replacement for clinical and radiographic response assessments in the future.

7. Richter's transformation

Maurice Richter initially described the transformation of CLL into an more aggressive form of lymphoma and since then this has been recognized as Richter's Transformation (RT) [67]. In most cases RT consists of transformation of CLL into Diffuse Large B Cell Lymphoma (DLBCL), however other aggressive lymphomas have been reported. As of now the reported incidence of RT in the era of novel agents is not very different from the incidence of RT in the chemoimmunotherapy era [68, 69] with incidence rates varying from 3–20% among various studies. RT is suspected when there is rapid clinical deterioration, worsening discordant lymphadenopathy to new onset cytopenia. However, its presentation can be varied. When RT is suspected a comprehensive evaluation with a PET/CT, image guided biopsy as well as a bone marrow biopsy is required. SUV of greater than 10 can distinguish RT form CLL with high sensitivity (91%) and specificity (95%) [70]. However, this has been disputed in the setting of novel agents and thus a concern for RT necessitates a biopsy of the index lesion preferably. RT primarily arises in the background of TP53 disruption and complex karyotype. MYC activation and CDKN2A/B likely play an important role in RT. Clonally related RT patients (>80% of RT DLBCL) respond very poorly to traditional chemotherapy for DLBCL, whereas clonally unrelated DLBCL RT patients respond to traditional chemotherapy just as de novo DLBCL. Thus, determination of clonal evolution is important but difficult to determine [71].Trials performed prior to the use of novel agents used R-CHOP or similar

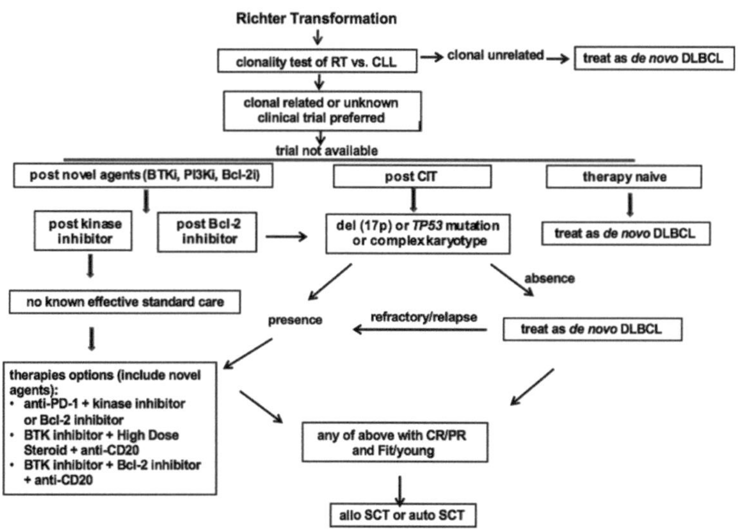

Figure 3.
Richter transformation. Adapted by ASH education handbook [73].

regimens as the standard therapy to treat RT. Fit patients who achieve a complete response or good partial response achieve benefit from a post induction strategy involving stem cell transplant [72]. Novel combinations, PDL-1 blockade and CAR-T or bispecific antibodies are being currently investigated as potential treatment options [72]. **Figure 3** below shows a suggested treatment approach algorithm for suspected patients with RT.

8. Hypogammaglobulinemia and autoimmune hemolytic anemia (AIHA)

8.1 CLL and hypogammaglobulinemia

Hypogammaglobulinemia is the most predominant inherent immune defect in CLL patients, with subtypes IgG3 and IgG4 particularly affected. Hypogammaglobulinemia becomes more pronounced with longer disease duration and advanced-stage disease. There is generally no reversal in this defect, even with response to therapy. However, in one report, ibrutinib therapy resulted in partial reconstitution of humoral immunity, with an increase in IgA levels [73]. The most common site of infection in CLL patients is the respiratory tract, which may be related to serum IgA and IgG4 deficiencies and possibly to mucosal immune defects. The majority of patients with CLL will develop hypogammaglobulinemia at some point in the course of their disease. The use of prophylactic intravenous immunoglobulin (IVIG) to restore IgG levels is controversial. For most patients with CLL, prophylactic IVIG is **not** recommended. For patients with CLL who have had recurrent infections requiring intravenous (IV) antibiotics or hospitalization and who also have a serum IgG <500 mg/dL, it is reasonable to administer IVIG. The usual dose is 200–400 mg/kg by IV infusion, given at three- to four-week intervals. The goal is to maintain the trough serum IgG in treated patients above 500–700 mg/dL as a general guideline. If there is a substantial decrease in the incidence of infections, treatment at gradually extended intervals may be considered. There is no good endpoint for when such therapy can be discontinued. The randomized trials of prophylactic IVIG found that patients who receive IVIG have a decreased incidence of minor and moderate, but not major, bacterial infections. However, IVIG does not appear to increase quality of life or survival [74]. Potential toxicities related to IVIG include anaphylaxis, fever, chills, "flu-like" symptoms, and headache. Another important aspect of IVIG therapy is that it replaces neither IgM nor IgA.

8.2 CLL and AIHA

CLL is frequently associated with autoimmune phenomena, the most common being autoimmune hemolytic anemia (AIHA) [75]. Up to 33% of CLL cases have a positive direct antiglobulin test (DAT) during the course of disease, but overt AIHA occurs much less frequently. In a report of 1203 patients with CLL consecutive cases reported from a single institution, 52 (4.3%) cases of AIHA were observed, 19 at the time of diagnosis [76]. The prevalence of AIHA in patients with CLL have been reported in the range of 4–10%. It increases with disease stage. The autoantibodies that cause AIHA can be produced by nonmalignant B cells or, less commonly, by the malignant CLL clone itself [77, 78]. In practice, AIHA may occur in patients with no other requirement for treatment, or in patients in whom chemotherapy treatment is imminent or already started. Factors associated with an increased risk of development of AIHA at diagnosis included a high white blood count, older age, and male sex. AIHA alone was not itself associated with poor prognosis. The diagnosis of

AIHA is usually based on the presence of an isolated fall in hemoglobin associated with a positive DAT, increased reticulocytes, and serum bilirubin. There have been no controlled trials of treatment for AIHA in CLL and the treatment approach is based on personal and institutional experience. In general, AIHA is responsive to CLL treatment, but if there is no indication to treat CLL, AIHA should be treated as a separate entity with steroids and other immune suppressants, the details of which is beyond the scope of this chapter. There has been controversy whether some chemotherapy agents, particularly purine analogs, induce or worsen AIHA. In a trial comparing outcomes of treatments using chlorambucil, fludarabine, or fludarabine in combination with cyclophosphamide, a positive DAT was found in 14%, and AIHA occurred in 10% of patients [75]. AIHA occurred more often in patients treated with chlorambucil than fludarabine, and occurred least frequently in patients receiving the combination of fludarabine and cyclophosphamide. For patients requiring therapy, a positive DAT test had poor prognostic significance, even in the absence of AIHA. The results suggest that the most successful treatment of AIHA in patients requiring chemotherapy treatment is the treatment associated with the best response rate.

9. Future directions

In summary, there has been a significant change in how we manage patients in CLL over the last 5 years. We have shifted away from chemoimmunotherapy towards novel agents such as BTK, PIK3, and BCL-2 inhibitors, which are not only more efficacious but are also safer and better tolerated. New prognostic models are being developed, and it appears that MRD directed therapy will become the norm in the future. Many clinical trials are looking at various combinations of novel therapies, with a defined period of treatment based on MRD analysis, to enable patients to have a period of treatment-free remission instead of continuous therapy.

Author details

Yazan Samhouri, Rupin Shah and Cyrus Khan
Department of Hematology and Cellular Therapy, Allegheny Health Network, West Penn Hospital, Pittsburgh, USA

*Address all correspondence to: clarasilvestr@gmail.com

References

[1] Jemal A, Siegel R, Ward E, Murray T, Xu J, Thun MJ. Cancer statistics, 2007. CA: A Cancer Journal for Clinicians. 2007;**57**(1):43-66

[2] Hallek M, Cheson BD, Catovsky D, Caligaris-Cappio F, Dighiero G, Dohner H, et al. iwCLL guidelines for diagnosis, indications for treatment, response assessment, and supportive management of CLL. Blood. 2018;**131**(25):2745-2760

[3] Campo E, Swerdlow SH, Harris NL, Pileri S, Stein H, Jaffe ES. The 2008 WHO classification of lymphoid neoplasms and beyond: Evolving concepts and practical applications. Blood. 2011;**117**(19):5019-5032

[4] Marti GE. The changing definition of CLL. Blood. 2009;**113**(18):4130-4131

[5] Hallek M, Cheson BD, Catovsky D, Caligaris-Cappio F, Dighiero G, Dohner H, et al. Guidelines for the diagnosis and treatment of chronic lymphocytic leukemia: A report from the international workshop on chronic lymphocytic leukemia updating the National Cancer Institute-working group 1996 guidelines. Blood. 2008;**111**(12):5446-5456

[6] Hansen MM. Chronic lymphocytic leukaemia. Clinical studies based on 189 cases followed for a long time. Scandinavian Journal of Haematology. Supplementum. 1973;**18**:3-286

[7] Galton DA. The pathogenesis of chronic lymphocytic leukemia. Canadian Medical Association Journal. 1966;**94**(19):1005-1010

[8] Boggs DR, Sofferman SA, Wintrobe MM, Cartwright GE. Factors influencing the duration of survival of patients with chronic lymphocytic leukemia. The American Journal of Medicine. 1966;**40**(2):243-254

[9] Chronic lymphocytic leukemia: Recommendations for diagnosis, staging, and response criteria. International workshop on chronic lymphocytic leukemia. Annals of Internal Medicine. 1989;**110**(3):236-238

[10] Call TG, Norman AD, Hanson CA, Achenbach SJ, Kay NE, Zent CS, et al. Incidence of chronic lymphocytic leukemia and high-count monoclonal B-cell lymphocytosis using the 2008 guidelines. Cancer. 2014;**120**(13):2000-2005

[11] Rai KR, Sawitsky A, Cronkite EP, Chanana AD, Levy RN, Pasternack BS. Clinical staging of chronic lymphocytic leukemia. Blood. 1975;**46**(2):219-234

[12] Keating MJ, Scouros M, Murphy S, Kantarjian H, Hester J, McCredie KB, et al. Multiple agent chemotherapy (POACH) in previously treated and untreated patients with chronic lymphocytic leukemia. Leukemia. 1988;**2**(3):157-164

[13] Binet JL, Leporrier M, Dighiero G, Charron D, D'Athis P, Vaugier G, et al. A clinical staging system for chronic lymphocytic leukemia: Prognostic significance. Cancer. 1977;**40**(2):855-864

[14] Zent CS, Ding W, Schwager SM, Reinalda MS, Hoyer JD, Jelinek DF, et al. The prognostic significance of cytopenia in chronic lymphocytic leukaemia/small lymphocytic lymphoma. British Journal of Haematology. 2008;**141**(5):615-621

[15] Moreno C, Hodgson K, Ferrer G, Elena M, Filella X, Pereira A, et al. Autoimmune cytopenia in chronic lymphocytic leukemia: Prevalence, clinical associations, and prognostic significance. Blood. 2010;**116**(23):4771-4776

[16] Muntañola A, Bosch F, Arguis P, Arellano-Rodrigo E, Ayuso C, Giné E, et al. Abdominal computed tomography predicts progression in patients with Rai stage 0 chronic lymphocytic leukemia. Journal of Clinical Oncology. 2007;**25**(12):1576-1580

[17] Rassenti LZ, Jain S, Keating MJ, Wierda WG, Grever MR, Byrd JC, et al. Relative value of ZAP-70, CD38, and immunoglobulin mutation status in predicting aggressive disease in chronic lymphocytic leukemia. Blood. 2008;**112**(5):1923-1930

[18] Molica S, Alberti A. Prognostic value of the lymphocyte doubling time in chronic lymphocytic leukemia. Cancer. 1987;**60**(11):2712-2716

[19] Wierda WG, O'Brien S, Wang X, Faderl S, Ferrajoli A, Do KA, et al. Characteristics associated with important clinical end points in patients with chronic lymphocytic leukemia at initial treatment. Journal of Clinical Oncology. 2009;**27**(10):1637-1643

[20] Damle RN, Wasil T, Fais F, Ghiotto F, Valetto A, Allen SL, et al. Ig V gene mutation status and CD38 expression as novel prognostic indicators in chronic lymphocytic leukemia. Blood. 1999;**94**(6):1840-1847

[21] An international prognostic index for patients with chronic lymphocytic leukaemia (CLL-IPI): A meta-analysis of individual patient data. The Lancet Oncology. 2016;**17**(6):779-790

[22] Knospe WH, Loeb V Jr, Huguley CM Jr. Bi-weekly chlorambucil treatment of chronic lymphocytic leukemia. Cancer. 1974;**33**(2):555-562

[23] Catovsky D, Else M, Richards S. Chlorambucil--still not bad: a reappraisal. Clinical Lymphoma, Myeloma & Leukemia. 2011;**11** (Suppl 1):S2-S6

[24] Johnson S, Smith AG, Loffler H, Osby E, Juliusson G, Emmerich B, et al. Multicentre prospective randomised trial of fludarabine versus cyclophosphamide, doxorubicin, and prednisone (CAP) for treatment of advanced-stage chronic lymphocytic leukaemia. The French cooperative group on CLL. Lancet (London, England). 1996;**347**(9013):1432-1438

[25] Rai KR, Peterson BL, Appelbaum FR, Kolitz J, Elias L, Shepherd L, et al. Fludarabine compared with chlorambucil as primary therapy for chronic lymphocytic leukemia. The New England Journal of Medicine. 2000;**343**(24):1750-1757

[26] Robak T, Blonski JZ, Kasznicki M, Konopka L, Ceglarek B, Dmoszynska A, et al. Cladribine with or without prednisone in the treatment of previously treated and untreated B-cell chronic lymphocytic leukaemia—Updated results of the multicentre study of 378 patients. British Journal of Haematology. 2000;**108**(2):357-368

[27] Robak T, Blonski JZ, Kasznicki M, Blasinska-Morawiec M, Krykowski E, Dmoszynska A, et al. Cladribine with prednisone versus chlorambucil with prednisone as first-line therapy in chronic lymphocytic leukemia: Report of a prospective, randomized, multicenter trial. Blood. 2000;**96**(8):2723-2729

[28] O'Brien SM, Kantarjian HM, Cortes J, Beran M, Koller CA, Giles FJ, et al. Results of the fludarabine and cyclophosphamide combination regimen in chronic lymphocytic leukemia. Journal of Clinical Oncology. 2001;**19**(5):1414-1420

[29] Keating MJ, O'Brien S, Albitar M, Lerner S, Plunkett W, Giles F, et al. Early results of a chemoimmunotherapy regimen of fludarabine, cyclophosphamide, and rituximab as initial therapy for chronic lymphocytic

leukemia. Journal of Clinical Oncology. 2005;**23**(18):4079-4088

[30] Thompson PA, Tam CS, O'Brien SM, Wierda WG, Stingo F, Plunkett W, et al. Fludarabine, cyclophosphamide, and rituximab treatment achieves long-term disease-free survival in IGHV-mutated chronic lymphocytic leukemia. Blood. 2016;**127**(3):303-309

[31] Hallek M, Fischer K, Fingerle-Rowson G, Fink AM, Busch R, Mayer J, et al. Addition of rituximab to fludarabine and cyclophosphamide in patients with chronic lymphocytic leukaemia: A randomised, open-label, phase 3 trial. Lancet (London, England). 2010;**376**(9747):1164-1174

[32] Fischer K, Bahlo J, Fink AM, Goede V, Herling CD, Cramer P, et al. Long-term remissions after FCR chemoimmunotherapy in previously untreated patients with CLL: Updated results of the CLL8 trial. Blood. 2016;**127**(2):208-215

[33] Fischer K, Cramer P, Stilgenbauer S, Busch R, Balleisen L, Kilp J, et al. Bendamustine combined with rituximab (BR) in first-line therapy of advanced CLL: A multicenter phase II trial of the German CLL study group (GCLLSG). Blood. 2009;**114**(22):205

[34] Michallet AS, Aktan M, Hiddemann W, Ilhan O, Johansson P, Laribi K, et al. Rituximab plus bendamustine or chlorambucil for chronic lymphocytic leukemia: Primary analysis of the randomized, open-label MABLE study. Haematologica. 2018;**103**(4):698-706

[35] Goede V, Fischer K, Bosch F, Follows G, Frederiksen H, Cuneo A, et al. Updated survival analysis from the CLL11 study: Obinutuzumab versus rituximab in Chemoimmunotherapy-treated patients with chronic lymphocytic leukemia. Blood. 2015;**126**(23):1733

[36] Hillmen P, Robak T, Janssens A, Babu KG, Kloczko J, Grosicki S, et al. Chlorambucil plus ofatumumab versus chlorambucil alone in previously untreated patients with chronic lymphocytic leukaemia (COMPLEMENT 1): A randomised, multicentre, open-label phase 3 trial. Lancet (London, England). 2015;**385**(9980):1873-1883

[37] Burger JA, Tedeschi A, Barr PM, Robak T, Owen C, Ghia P, et al. Ibrutinib as initial therapy for patients with chronic lymphocytic leukemia. New England Journal of Medicine. 2015;**373**(25):2425-2437

[38] Shanafelt TD, Wang V, Kay NE, Hanson CA, O'Brien SM, Barrientos JC, et al. A randomized phase III study of ibrutinib (PCI-32765)-based therapy vs. standard fludarabine, cyclophosphamide, and rituximab (FCR) chemoimmunotherapy in untreated younger patients with chronic lymphocytic leukemia (CLL): A trial of the ECOG-ACRIN cancer research group (E1912). The American Society of Hematology. 2018

[39] Woyach JA, Ruppert AS, Heerema NA, Zhao W, Booth AM, Ding W, et al. Ibrutinib alone or in combination with rituximab produces superior progression free survival (PFS) compared with Bendamustine plus rituximab in untreated older patients with chronic lymphocytic leukemia (cll): Results of alliance north american intergroup study A041202. The American Society of Hematology. 2018

[40] Moreno C, Greil R, Demirkan F, Tedeschi A, Anz B, Larratt L, et al. Ibrutinib + Obinutuzumab versus Chlorambucil + Obinutuzumab As first-line treatment in patients with chronic lymphocytic leukemia or small lymphocytic lymphoma (CLL/SLL): Results from phase 3 iLLUMINATE. Blood. 2018;**132**(Suppl 1):691

[41] Ahn IE, Farooqui MZH, Tian X, Valdez J, Sun C, Soto S, et al. Depth and durability of response to ibrutinib in CLL: 5-year follow-up of a phase 2 study. Blood. 2018;**131**(21):2357-2366

[42] Ahn IE, Farber CM, Davids MS, Grinblatt DL, Kay NE, Lamanna N, et al. Early progression of disease as a predictor of survival in chronic lymphocytic leukemia. Blood Advances. 2017;**1**(25):2433-2443

[43] Seymour JF, Robertson LE, O'Brien S, Lerner S, Keating MJ. Survival of young patients with chronic lymphocytic leukemia failing fludarabine therapy: A basis for the use of myeloablative therapies. Leukemia & Lymphoma. 1995;**18**(5-6):493-496

[44] Herman SE, Gordon AL, Hertlein E, Ramanunni A, Zhang X, Jaglowski S, et al. Bruton tyrosine kinase represents a promising therapeutic target for treatment of chronic lymphocytic leukemia and is effectively targeted by PCI-32765. Blood. 2011;**117**(23):6287-6296

[45] Byrd JC, Brown JR, O'Brien S, Barrientos JC, Kay NE, Reddy NM, et al. Ibrutinib versus ofatumumab in previously treated chronic lymphoid leukemia. The New England Journal of Medicine. 2014;**371**(3):213-223

[46] O'Brien S, Jones JA, Coutre SE, Mato AR, Hillmen P, Tam C, et al. Ibrutinib for patients with relapsed or refractory chronic lymphocytic leukaemia with 17p deletion (RESONATE-17): A phase 2, open-label, multicentre study. The Lancet Oncology. 2016;**17**(10):1409-1418

[47] Brown JR, Moslehi J, O'Brien S, Ghia P, Hillmen P, Cymbalista F, et al. Characterization of atrial fibrillation adverse events reported in ibrutinib randomized controlled registration trials. Haematologica. 2017;**102**(10):1796-1805

[48] Lipsky AH, Farooqui MZ, Tian X, Martyr S, Cullinane AM, Nghiem K, et al. Incidence and risk factors of bleeding-related adverse events in patients with chronic lymphocytic leukemia treated with ibrutinib. Haematologica. 2015;**100**(12):1571-1578

[49] Furman RR, Sharman JP, Coutre SE, Cheson BD, Pagel JM, Hillmen P, et al. Idelalisib and rituximab in relapsed chronic lymphocytic leukemia. The New England Journal of Medicine. 2014;**370**(11):997-1007

[50] Zelenetz AD, Barrientos JC, Brown JR, Coiffier B, Delgado J, Egyed M, et al. Idelalisib or placebo in combination with bendamustine and rituximab in patients with relapsed or refractory chronic lymphocytic leukaemia: Interim results from a phase 3, randomised, double-blind, placebo-controlled trial. The Lancet Oncology. 2017;**18**(3):297-311

[51] Jones JA, Robak T, Brown JR, Awan FT, Badoux X, Coutre S, et al. Efficacy and safety of idelalisib in combination with ofatumumab for previously treated chronic lymphocytic leukaemia: An open-label, randomised phase 3 trial. The Lancet Haematology. 2017;**4**(3):e114-ee26

[52] Flinn IW, Hillmen P, Montillo M, Nagy Z, Illes A, Etienne G, et al. The phase 3 DUO trial: Duvelisib vs ofatumumab in relapsed and refractory CLL/SLL. Blood. 2018;**132**(23):2446-2455

[53] Stilgenbauer S, Eichhorst B, Schetelig J, Coutre S, Seymour JF, Munir T, et al. Venetoclax in relapsed or refractory chronic lymphocytic leukaemia with 17p deletion: A multicentre, open-label, phase 2 study. The Lancet Oncology. 2016;**17**(6):768-778

[54] Jones JA, Mato AR, Wierda WG, Davids MS, Choi M, Cheson BD, et al.

Venetoclax for chronic lymphocytic leukaemia progressing after ibrutinib: An interim analysis of a multicentre, open-label, phase 2 trial. The Lancet Oncology. 2018;**19**(1):65-75

[55] Seymour JF, Kipps TJ, Eichhorst B, Hillmen P, D'Rozario J, Assouline S, et al. Venetoclax-rituximab in relapsed or refractory chronic lymphocytic leukemia. The New England Journal of Medicine. 2018;**378**(12):1107-1120

[56] Tam CS, O'Brien S, Plunkett W, Wierda W, Ferrajoli A, Wang X, et al. Long-term results of first salvage treatment in CLL patients treated initially with FCR (fludarabine, cyclophosphamide, rituximab). Blood. 2014;**124**(20):3059-3064

[57] Eichhorst B, Fink AM, Bahlo J, Busch R, Kovacs G, Maurer C, et al. First-line chemoimmunotherapy with bendamustine and rituximab versus fludarabine, cyclophosphamide, and rituximab in patients with advanced chronic lymphocytic leukaemia (CLL10): An international, open-label, randomised, phase 3, non-inferiority trial. The Lancet Oncology. 2016;**17**(7):928-942

[58] Knauf WU, Lissichkov T, Aldaoud A, Liberati A, Loscertales J, Herbrecht R, et al. Phase III randomized study of bendamustine compared with chlorambucil in previously untreated patients with chronic lymphocytic leukemia. Journal of Clinical Oncology. 2009;**27**(26):4378-4384

[59] Wierda WG, Kipps TJ, Mayer J, Stilgenbauer S, Williams CD, Hellmann A, et al. Ofatumumab as single-agent CD20 immunotherapy in fludarabine-refractory chronic lymphocytic leukemia. Journal of Clinical Oncology. 2010;**28**(10):1749-1755

[60] Khouri IF, Keating M, Korbling M, Przepiorka D, Anderlini P, O'Brien S, et al. Transplant-lite: Induction of graft-versus-malignancy using fludarabine-based nonablative chemotherapy and allogeneic blood progenitor-cell transplantation as treatment for lymphoid malignancies. Journal of Clinical Oncology. 1998;**16**(8):2817-2824

[61] Sorror ML, Storer BE, Maloney DG, Sandmaier BM, Martin PJ, Storb R. Outcomes after allogeneic hematopoietic cell transplantation with nonmyeloablative or myeloablative conditioning regimens for treatment of lymphoma and chronic lymphocytic leukemia. Blood 2008;111(1):446-452.

[62] Dreger P, Schnaiter A, Zenz T, Böttcher S, Rossi M, Paschka P, et al. TP53, SF3B1, and NOTCH1 mutations and outcome of allotransplantation for chronic lymphocytic leukemia: Six-year follow-up of the GCLLSG CLL3X trial. Blood. 2013;**121**(16):3284-3288

[63] van Gelder M, de Wreede LC, Bornhauser M, Niederwieser D, Karas M, Anderson NS, et al. Long-term survival of patients with CLL after allogeneic transplantation: A report from the European Society for Blood and Marrow Transplantation. Bone Marrow Transplantation. 2017;**52**(3):372-380

[64] Bottcher S, Ritgen M, Fischer K, Stilgenbauer S, Busch RM, Fingerle-Rowson G, et al. Minimal residual disease quantification is an independent predictor of progression-free and overall survival in chronic lymphocytic leukemia: A multivariate analysis from the randomized GCLLSG CLL8 trial. Journal of Clinical Oncology. 2012;**30**(9):980-988

[65] Gribben JG. How and when I do allogeneic transplant in CLL. Blood. 2018;**132**(1):31-39

[66] O'Brien S, Furman RR, Coutre S, Flinn IW, Burger JA, Blum K, et al. Single-agent ibrutinib in

treatment-naive and relapsed/refractory chronic lymphocytic leukemia: A 5-year experience. Blood. 2018;**131**(17):1910-1919

[67] Richter MN. Generalized reticular cell sarcoma of lymph nodes associated with lymphatic leukemia. The American Journal of Pathology. 1928;**4**(4):285-92.7

[68] Maurer C, Langerbeins P, Bahlo J, Cramer P, Fink AM, Pflug N, et al. Effect of first-line treatment on second primary malignancies and Richter's transformation in patients with CLL. Leukemia. 2016;**30**(10):2019-2025

[69] Maddocks KJ, Ruppert AS, Lozanski G, Heerema NA, Zhao W, Abruzzo L, et al. Etiology of Ibrutinib therapy discontinuation and outcomes in patients with chronic lymphocytic leukemia. JAMA Oncology. 2015;**1**(1):80-87

[70] Michallet A-S, Sesques P, Rabe KG, Itti E, Tordot J, Tychyj-Pinel C, et al. An 18F-FDG-PET maximum standardized uptake value > 10 represents a novel valid marker for discerning Richter's syndrome. Leukemia & Lymphoma. 2016;**57**(6):1474-1477

[71] Rossi D, Spina V, Deambrogi C, Rasi S, Laurenti L, Stamatopoulos K, et al. The genetics of Richter syndrome reveals disease heterogeneity and predicts survival after transformation. Blood. 2011;**117**(12):3391-3401

[72] Ding W. Richter transformation in the era of novel agents. Hematology. American Society of Hematology. Education Program. 2018;**2018**(1):256-263

[73] Sun C, Tian X, Lee YS, Gunti S, Lipsky A, Herman SE, et al. Partial reconstitution of humoral immunity and fewer infections in patients with chronic lymphocytic leukemia treated with ibrutinib. Blood. 2015;**126**(19):2213-2219

[74] Gale RP, Chapel HM, Bunch C, Rai KR, Foon K, Courter SG, et al. Intravenous immunoglobulin for the prevention of infection in chronic lymphocytic leukemia. A randomized, controlled clinical trial. The New England Journal of Medicine. 1988;**319**(14):902-907

[75] Dearden C, Wade R, Else M, Richards S, Milligan D, Hamblin T, et al. The prognostic significance of a positive direct antiglobulin test in chronic lymphocytic leukemia: A beneficial effect of the combination of fludarabine and cyclophosphamide on the incidence of hemolytic anemia. Blood. 2008;**111**(4):1820-1826

[76] Mauro FR, Foa R, Cerretti R, Giannarelli D, Coluzzi S, Mandelli F, et al. Autoimmune hemolytic anemia in chronic lymphocytic leukemia: Clinical, therapeutic, and prognostic features. Blood. 2000;**95**(9):2786-2792

[77] Duhrsen U, Augener W, Zwingers T, Brittinger G. Spectrum and frequency of autoimmune derangements in lymphoproliferative disorders: Analysis of 637 cases and comparison with myeloproliferative diseases. British Journal of Haematology. 1987;**67**(2):235-239

[78] Visco C, Barcellini W, Maura F, Neri A, Cortelezzi A, Rodeghiero F. Autoimmune cytopenias in chronic lymphocytic leukemia. American Journal of Hematology. 2014;**89**(11):1055-1062

Chapter 7

Target Therapy in Hematological Malignancies

Safa Shukry, Fadhel Hariri and Abdul Wahab Al-Nehmi

Abstract

Molecular target therapy is a recently rapid progress in the management of hematological malignancies. In myeloid neoplasm, the sensational response to treatment and the overall survival and quality of life improvement for treatment with *tyrosine kinase inhibitors (TKI)* agents for patients with chronic myeloid leukemia and the introduction of Janus kinase (JAK)-2 inhibitors (ruxolitinib) may offer comparative advantage in myeloproliferative diseases of patients with polycythemia vera (PV), primary *myelofibrosis* (MF) and essential thrombocythemia (ET). The introduction of all-trans-retinoic acid (ATRA) and mylotarg for acute myeloid leukemia patients, have had major impacts on the treatment protocol plan and different other targeted therapeutic highly effective agents, including FLT3, histone deacetylase inhibitors and farnesyl transferase. In malignant lymphomas and lymphatic leukemia the feature has been the presentation of rituximab, with critical enhancements within the treatment of chronic lymphocytic leukemia and non-Hodgkin's lymphoma. The most recent 15 years has encountered a rapidly broadening interest and acknowledgment that leukemic stem cells, including an enhanced capacity to target them, may hold the way to enhanced reaction and diminished relapse rates over both lymphoid and myeloid disorders. Technical regulation for growing new personalized anticancer target therapy agents have changed and presently evaluated and screened.

Keywords: target therapy, hematological malignancy, leukemia, lymphoma, myeloma

1. Introduction

The past few a long time have seen gigantic changes within inside the approach to making advanced anticancer therapy, in one side due to advanced unused innovations and computer instruments, and on other side due to other ways of inquire about centered on progressing our understanding about the fundamental of molecular pathways and genetic changes that driving the advancement of cancer, discoveries which are making a difference us to superior distinguish which patients will advantage from the plan focused on treatment and permit the researcher to personalized target therapy guidelines. This ever-growing information base has too driven to the distinguishing proof of more molecular targets and the ensuing development of new focused on target therapy agents that will shaping treatment of cancer in the future [1].

Personalized targeted therapy is a drug that squares the cancer cells development by interfering with particular molecule needed for carcinogenesis and growth of tumors [2] instead of essentially interfering with quickly isolating dividing cells. The personalized target therapy for cancer diseases has been a noteworthy stimulus for the advancing field of pharmacogenomics. Moreover it is characterized as pharmacogenomics can envelop germline and significant (infection) gene and protein estimations utilized to expect the probability that a patient's tumor will react to an explicit single-agent or multiagent chemotherapy protocols and the chance of hurtful side effects [3]. Besides the *US Food and Drug Administration* (FDA) has considered target treatment as a personalized therapy approved and named with a specific reference to at the same time or as of now asserted illustrative test that must be performed some time recently the persistent can be considered qualified to get the target therapy agents [4].

Personalized targeted therapy begun modern transformation approximately the improvement of cancer treatment to a person patient's tumor, the financial matters of cancer care around the world. As expanded of analyzed patients with cancer and as these patients live longer, essential care clinics will make strides wellbeing care for patients who have gotten cancer target therapy [5, 6].

2. Development of target therapy

The outcome after revolution of target therapy was improved in lymphoma, myeloma and chronic leukemia. Imatinib as first generation of TKI has had an excellent outcome on chronic myeloid leukemia, bortezomib and rituximab, which has also high percentage of remission in myeloma and lymphoma, respectively [7, 8]. In patients with multiple myeloma preclinical studies have informed the rational use of combination therapies, such as bortezomib with lenalidomide to trigger both intrinsic and extrinsic apoptotic signaling [9].

Chronic lymphocytic leukemia (CLL), non-Hodgkin's lymphoma (NHL) and idiopathic myelofibrosis (IM) fundamentally influence elderly patients, numerous of whom have therapeutic comorbidities that constrain the utilize of standard chemotherapy. Treatment with target therapy such as imatinib and rituximab are frequently less harmful and superior endured than conventional chemotherapy, advertising these patients extra treatment choices [10].

3. Acute myeloid leukemia (AML)

The targeted therapy for patients with AML in recent years maybe most outstanding within the molecularly targeted *therapy* against its *specific* genetic abnormality of acute promyelocytic leukemia (APL). The initial (induction) *treatment of APL* with all-trans-retinoic acid (ATRA) play role in cells differentiation in patients with APL with *t(15;17)*(q22;q21) and has driven to disease-free survival and/or cure in 75% of patients with APL [11].

The introduction of ATRA in patients works to differentiation blast of acute promyelocytic leukemia (APL) to AML blast. The retinoic acid disorder is the most common complication characterized by fever, disseminated intravascular coagulation and cardiac, respiratory and renal function disorders. These disorders, which are seen in some patients, particularly patients associated with leukocytosis, can be treated or improved with chemotherapy or corticosteroids.

The current standard treatment of APL in induction and consolidation, include introduction of ATRA simultaneously with cytarabine and anthracycline and pursued by maintenance in combination with low-dose chemotherapy [12, 13].

Moreover, in an endeavor to maintain a strategic distance from routine chemotherapy, the addition of ATRA in combination with gemtuzumab ozogamicin has been utilized as induction with achievement of remissions (**Table 1**) [14]. Gemtuzumab ozogamicin (GO; Mylotarg) is a selective anti CD33 anti-body conjugated with calicheamicin facilitated against CD33 surface marker and communicated by more than 90% of myeloid leukemic blasts and is harmful to DNA calicheamicin. The overall response (OR) rate reported in 30% patients with AML and CD33+ treated with GO.

The rate of myelosuppression as common side effects of chemotherapy, was less with GO, in spite of the fact that acute *respiratory distress syndrome* and pulmonary edema have been experienced in patients with leukocytosis but less than 30,000/mL [15]. In May 2000, FDA have approved "GO" for patients above 60 years and after relapsing or for patients not fit for intensive chemotherapy [15–19]. On September 1, 2017, the (FDA) also approved "GO" for adult patients newly diagnosed AML with CD33+.

Ulocuplumab (BMS-936564/MDX-1338) may be a monoclonal antibodies agent which inhibits the official of the CXC chemokine receptor 4 (CXCR4) to fortify relocation from the bone marrow to peripheral blood stromal cell-derived chemokine CXC theme ligand 12 (CXCL12). In patients with refractory and relapsed AML, ulocuplumab in combination with mitoxantrone, etoposide and cytarabine driven to CR with partial recovery of bone marrow cell lines (CRi) in 51% patients studied [20].

The mutations of FLT 3 appear to be free destitute prognosticators in AML. The *Mutation in FLT3 gene* (FMS-like tyrosine kinase-3) occurs in 30% of FLT3-ITD and 7% of FLT3-TDK with AML. The FLT3 kinase inhibitors may be divided into 1st- and 2nd-generation drugs. 1st-generation: sorafenib, sunitinib, estaurtinib, midostaurin l, tandutinib, pacritinib; 2nd-generation: gliteritinib, quizartinib, crenolamid, ponatinib, JH-IX-179, PLX3397. The mutated *FLT3* gene has variable affectability according to type of target therapy [21].

Isocitrate dehydrogenase (IDH) takes place in lipid metabolism and the Krebs cycle, and it catalyzes the change of isocitrate to α-ketoglutarate. In AML the gene mutations IDH1 occur in 11% and IDH2 in 12% of cases. Enasidenib (AG-221/CC-90007) is the first single-agent selective IDH2 inhibitor to induce the differentiation of leukemic cells and orally well tolerated. AML in patients with refractory or relapsed with mutant-*IDH2* induced hematologic responses, and have more than 9 months median survival reported after treatment with Enasidenib [22].

Target	Drug	Group
CD33	Gemtuzumab ozogamycin, lintuzumab, vadastuximab talirine	High molecular mass drugs
CD33, CD3	AMG 330	
FLT3	1st-generation: sorafenib, midostaurin, lestaurtinib, sunitinib, tandutinib, pacritinib 2nd-generation: quizartinib, crenolamid, ponatinib, PLX3397, gliteritinib, JH-IX-179	Tyrosine kinase inhibitors
IDH	Cenasidenib	Cell pathway Inhibitors
BCL2	Navitoclax, venetoclax	
Topoisomerase II	Vosaroxin	
LSD1	ORY-1001, GSK2879552	Epigenetic modulators
HDAC	Pabinostat, vorinostat	

Table 1.
Targeted drugs in AML treatment.

Navitoclax is BCL2 inhibitor by ABT-199 with multiple anti-apoptotic of AML. Its antitumor activity is restricted by adverse effects, which is registered by the FDA for treating chronic lymphocytic leukemia (CLL) and AML [23].

Vosaroxin could be a topoisomerase II inhibitor which is one of the important randomized trials exploring therapeutic options for refractory and relapsed AML to date and considered basic for cell survival. Vosaroxin induces DNA destruction and is most successful among elderly patients more than 60 years of age with myelodysplastic disorder (MDS) or acute myeloid leukemia (AML) [24].

Lysine-specific demethylase 1 (LSD1) is a histone demethylase. LSD1 inhibition leads to the inhibition of growth and metastasis of tumor and also regulates the differentiation of stem cells and has potential novel treatment in acute myeloid leukemia (AML).

Panobinostat (LBH589) induces AML cell apoptosis in vitro by inhibiting the expression of repair proteins (e.g., BRCA1, CHK1 and RAD51), increasing the efficiency of cytarabine and daunorubicin, and it is promising in t(8;21) AML due to the pathological AML1/ETO protein that recruits histone deacetylases and in combination with Azacitidine (AZA) doubled the rate of response in high risk patients with CMML, MDS or AML not candidate for stem cell transplantation [25].

Vorinostat (suberoylanilidehydroxamic acid [SAHA]) advances cell cycle inhibition of growth and induces differentiation and cell apoptosis of AML and reported favorable overall survival in AML patients with FLT3 ITD mutations [26].

4. Acute lymphoblastic leukemia (ALL)

The classical main treatment for adult acute lymphoblastic leukemia (ALL) is *chemotherapy* drugs and in some patients the transplant of stem cells in adult patients has good results. Advance enhancement maybe calls for a diverse approach from conventional chemotherapy, such as target drugs with TKI (imatinib) and/or immunotherapy.

ALL with Philadelphia chromosome-positive (Ph+) have been noted with impressive response to intensive chemotherapy and imatinib [27].

CD20 is a B cell-specific surface antigen on mature B-ALL and precursor B-ALL, as well as in lymphoblastic lymphoma, would manage the probability of rituximab response. The introduction of target therapy (rituximab) in combination with chemotherapy (Hyper-CVAD) (rituximab with hyperfractionated cyclophosphamide, doxorubicin, vincristine and dexamethasone) in lymphoma or leukemia, reported complete remission rate of 90% with minimal toxicity [28, 29].

Acute lymphoblastic leukemia blast cells express specific antigens for CD22 in 90% of patients and have amazing clinical action indeed among intensely before treatment of elderly B-ALL patients and refractory and relapsed B-ALL patients after treatment with inotuzumab ozogamicin. Combination of inotuzumab ozogamicin with other treatments after chemotherapy may too possibly improve clinical outcomes [30].

Blinatumomab: is a CD3 and CD19-directed, to activate a B-cell specific inflammatory and cytolytic response. In 2006 FDA approved Blinatumomab for refractory and relapsed ALL [31]. Blinatumomab activates endogenous T cells by connecting CD19 on benign and malignant B cells with CD3 in the T-cell receptor complex in combination with chemotherapy or as single agents, in preclinical and clinical settings have produced varying response to induce tumor cell lysis via complement-dependent cytotoxicity or with antibody, induce cell death [32, 33].

5. Chronic myeloid (*Myelogenous*) leukemia (CML)

Chronic *Myelogenous* Leukemia (CML) is a clonal myeloproliferative disorder characterized by the increased and unregulated growth of *myeloid* cells due to translocation between long arms of chromosomes 9 and 22t (9;22) that generates tyrosine kinase BCR-ABL1 [34]. CML classified into 3 phases; chronic stable phase (CP) which the myeloid cell series is expanded but cellular differentiation is maintained and effortlessly controlled with treatment for a period that can last for 36–60 months but the accelerated phase (AP) can lasts for less than 12 months. Blast phase (BP) are still poorly understood, characterized by rapid expansion of myeloid or lymphoid with presence of more than 20% blast cells in the peripheral blood or bone marrow resulting in manifestation of ALL or AML and death in short period within 4–6 months [35].

Chronic myeloid (*Myelogenous)* leukemia treatment progressed significantly through the advancement of tyrosine kinase inhibitors (TKIs), particularly the presentation of imatinib into the clinical use. Imatinib is the drug of choice of the first generation in the chronic phase of CML and considered the golden standard target therapy in CML. The second generations also currently available for clinical use include nilotinib, dasatinib, bosutinib and ponatinib.

To maintain patients in remission and prevent progression of disease into accelerated and blast phases are the main treatment goals of chronic myeloid leukemias and keep the patients free of complications and with minimal drug related toxicity.

Target therapy with TKIs and allogenic bone marrow transplantation, play important role in improvement curative percentage of CML patients.

5.1 Imatinib (Gleevec)

Imatinib mesylate (IM), a phenylaminopyrimidine TKI that is the first drug of its class characterized by BCR-ABL TKI has excellent changes in the strategy of treatment of CML in the last 20 years. In May 2001, FDA has approved imatinib for the treatment of CML patients. Arthralgia, myalgia, nausea, and fluid retention are the common side effects in imatinib. About 97% complete hematologic response and 83% cytogenetic response was documented after many years of regular follow up of CML patients received imatinib [36, 37]. Patients with hematological or cytogenetic resistance to standard dosage of imatinib (400 mg) were begun with tall dosage (600–800 mg). Some of patients are unlikely to be overcome by high doses due to some specific mutations, in these cases alternative target therapy should be considered for patients fails or with suboptimal response [38].

5.2 Dasatinib (Sprycel)

Dasatinib is approved in 2006 as a kinase inhibitor of thiazole carboximide agent and molecular formula $C_{22}H_{26}ClN_7O_2S.H_2O$ with highly powerful dual Abl/Src kinase inhibitor against most imatinib-resistant mutants. Dasatinib considering the excellent treatment option for CML cases in chronic phase and other CML phases who develop resistance or fails response to imatinib and for cases with Ph+ALL [39]. Dasatinib is more than 300 times as powerful as imatinib in restraining unmutated BCR-ABL transcripts in vitro. The incidence of resistance to dasatinib is less than other TKI and the disease progression may be reduced among CML cases treated with dasatinib [40].

5.3 Nilotinib (Tasigna)

Nilotinib is a small molecule tyrosine kinase inhibitor in the form of hydrochloride monohydrate salt and is 20–30 times as potent as imatinib and can be replaced instead of imatinib. In 2007 nilotinib approved by (FDA) for utilize as a particular treatment for *Philadelphia chromosome-positive CML (Ph+CML).* Nilotinib was statistically superior in both complete cytogenetic response (CCyR) and major molecular response (MMR) ($p < 0.001$) [41].

5.4 Bosutinib (Bosulif)

FDA approved bosutinib in September 2012, for adult patients with all phases of chronic myeloid leukemia confirmed positive BCR-ABL. Bosutinib is an oral double ABL/SRC kinase inhibitor that is dynamic against numerous BCR-ABL transformations related with imatinib resistance. Bosutinib had the lowest rates of severe side effects, except for diarrhea. In especially, severe cardiovascular side effects were significantly less common in the bosutinib. They experience not complicated to develop blast crisis and progress to accelerated phase in 4% of cases. The overall survival at 2 years were 97% [42].

The suggested dosage of bosutinib is 500 mg oral daily dose with nourishment. The treatment will be proceeded concurring to plan take after up until progression of disease or intolerance of drug.

5.5 Ponatinib (Iclusig)

Ponatinib is approved in December 2012 by the US-FDA as a third generation TKI. Ponatinib is indicated for all phases of CML patients develop resistant to nilotinib or dasatinib or not tolerate to nilotinib or dasatinib and for ALL patients with Philadelphia chromosome positive and resistant to imatinib, dasatinib or nilotinib.

Patients with severely leukocytosis and patients with monocytosis, are less response to tyrosine kinase inhibitors, and have a higher risk of transformation to accelerated and blast phase [43]. The dose of ponatinib recommended daily is 45 mg with modification according to side effects. The recommendations for treatment of CML according to European LeukemiaNet summarized in **Table 2**.

5.6 Monitoring therapeutic response in CML

The target treatment checking can be performing concurring to inquire about laboratory recommendations for scoring molecular response by utilizing either a cytogenetic or molecular tests, or both, depending on the open facilities. The molecular response to TKI treatment of patients with CML is exceptionally imperative component of CML management with standard take after up each 3 months agreeing to ELN guidelines to realize early molecular response playing an imperative part in helpful decision making (**Table 3**) [45].

The TKI response is the foremost vital prognostic figure. The forecast for CML patients in accelerated and blast phases (AP and BP) is less than that seen in chronic stage (CP). The treatment responses are characterized as optimal, suboptimal or failure. Complete remission accomplished with optimal response which is the most excellent result comparable with that of the common populace. Failure implies that the understanding ought to get a distinctive treatment to restrain the chance of progression of disease and death [46]. Fractional abatement or the problematic response is the intermediate zone between optimal response and failure and usually considered as “warning” for moving to moment line TKI **Table 3**.

First line	Imatinib (400 mg daily) or nilotinib (300 mg twice daily) or dasatinib (100 mg daily)
	HLA type patients and siblings only in case of baseline warnings (high risk, major route CCA/Ph+)
2nd line, intolerance to the first TKI	Anyone of the other TKIs approved first line (imatinib 400 mg twice daily, nilotinib 400 mg twice daily, dasatinib (70 mg twice daily)
Second line, failure of imatinib first line	Dasatinib or nilotinib or bosutinib 500 mg daily or ponatinib (45 mg daily)
	HLA type patients and siblings
2nd line, failure of nilotinib first line	Bosutinib or dasatinib or ponatinib; search for an unrelated stem cell donor; consider AlloSCT and prepare HLA type patients and siblings
2nd line, dasatinib failure as first line	Bosutinib or Nilotinib or ponatinib
	HLA type patients and siblings; search for an unrelated stem cell donor; consider AlloSCT
3rd line, intolerance or failure to 2 TKIs	Anyone of the remaining TKIs; alloSCT recommended in all eligible patients
Any line, T315I mutation	Ponatinib/omacitaxine; consider AlloSCT and search for an unrelated stem cell donor

CCA/Ph+; clonal chromosome abnormalities in Ph+ cells, alloSCT; allogenic stem cell transplantation.

Table 2.
Target therapy recommendations for chronic myeloid leukemia modified of Abdul Hamid et al. [34].

Complete hematological response (CHR): complete blood counts normalization and spleen return to normal with disappearance of chronic myeloid leukemia (CML) manifestations
Complete cytogenetic response (CCyR): absence of Philadelphia chromosome (Ph) in 20 of 20 bone marrow metaphases by karyotyping.
Major cytogenetic response (MCyR): presence of Philadelphia chromosome in 0–35% of 20 metaphases.
Molecular response: by follow up of quantitative real time PCR (qRT-PCR) analysis, the *BCR-ABL1*/control gene transcript ratio is determined using the International Scale (IS) standardized baseline. $\geq 3\log_{10}$ reduction in *BCR-ABL1* transcripts ($\leq$0.10% IS) is major molecular response (MMR).
Optimal response: complete hematological response (CHR) and $\leq$65% Ph+ metaphases at 3 months of imatinib therapy, $\leq$35% Ph+ metaphases at 6 months, CCyR at 12 months and MMR at 18 months.
Suboptimal response: There is no fulfilling criteria for either optimal response or failure. The suboptimal response according to ELN recommendations implies that the long term benefits of imatinib are doubtful.
Failure: There is no complete hematological response at 3 months of imatinib therapy, >95% Ph+ metaphases at 6 months, >35% Ph+ metaphases at 12 months and no MMR at 18 months. Absence of CHR, BCR-ABL1 mutations, clonal cytogenetic evolution, define failure at any time during treatment.

Table 3.
Criteria of therapeutic response [44].

6. Chronic lymphocytic leukemia (CLL)

Chronic lymphocytic leukemia (chronic lymphoid leukemia CLL), is a heterogeneous disease characterized by the proliferation of functionally incompetent in the peripheral blood, bone marrow, spleen and lymph nodes. CLL is a disease of adult the elder age group as with a median onset at initial diagnosis of 70 and 75 years old and the male to female ratio 2:1 [47].

6.1 Treatment of chronic lymphoyctic leukemia

The CLL disease extent and prognosis according to Rai and Binet staging systems. Early stages (0, I, II) and symptomatic patient keep for observation and regular follow up without treatment. 70% of CLL patients respond to chlorambucil monotherapy which may be given orally for stabilization of leukocytosis and symptoms. Thrombocytopenia in stage IV stabilized with addition of prednisone.

6.2 Purine nucleoside analogous: (fludarabin, deoxycoformycin, 2-chlorodeoxy-adenosine)

Are unique drugs that are effective in low grade lymphomas and chronic lymphatic leukemia.

Fludarabine is active and useful in patients resist to chlorambucil and in newly diagnosed CLL. The alternative use of CVP (Cyclophosphamide, Vincristine and Prednisone). In addition fludarabine and cladribine in treatment of CLL, the combination of rituximab against CD20 and alemtuzumab against CD52, has an acceptable safety profile, and has clinical activity with a short course in patients with refractory or relapsed to chemotherapy.

6.3 Ibrutinib (Imbruvica)

Is a small molecule targeted drug that acts as an irreversible burton tyrosine kinase inhibitor (BTK) and can be used to treat chronic lymphocytic leukemia (CLL). In 2013 FDA approved ibrutinib for treatment patients with mantle cell lymphoma and in 2013 also approved for CLL and small lymphocytic lymphoma with 17p [48, 49].

6.4 Idelalisib (Zydelig)

Is another targeted drug approved for patients with CLL with CD20 positive in combination with rituximab or ofatumumab. It blocks a kinase protein called PI3K. FDA in July 28, 2014, has approved idelalisib 150 mg tablets for the treatment of B-CLL. Idelalisib has been appeared to assist treat CLL after other medications have been attempted and is indicated in combination with rituximab for patients with relapsed chronic lymphocytic leukemia (CLL) and significantly reported excellent response rate, overall survival and progressed progression-free survival (**Tables 4** and **5**) [50, 51].

6.5 Venetoclax (Venclexta)

Is a selective drug that targets BCL-2, a protein in CLL cells had a manageable response for patients with small lymphocytic lymphoma (SLL) poor prognostic and chronic lymphocytic leukemia whose relapsed or refractory to other drugs (**Tables 4** and **5**) [52].

Mechanism	Drug	Target
Monoclonal antibodies	MEDI-551	CD19
	Ofatumumab	CD20
	Obinutuzumab	CD20
	Epratuzumab	CD22
	Lucatumumab	CD40
Antibody drug conjugates	Brentuximab vedotin	CD30
	Polatuzumab vedotin	CD79B
	Inotuzumab ozogamicin	CD22
	SAR3419	CD19

Table 4.
Novel antibodies and antibody-drug conjugates directed against surface antigens [49].

Mechanism	Drug	Target
Immune checkpoint inhibitors	Ipilimumab	CTLA-4
	Pidilizumab	PD-1
	Nivolumab	PD-1
	Pembrolizumab	PD-1
Small molecule inhibitors	Ibrutinib	BTK
	Idelalisib	PI3Kd
	Duvelisib	PI3Kgd
	Copanlisib	PI3Kd
	Navitoclax	Bcl-2
	Venetoclax	Bcl-2

Table 5.
Novel antibodies directed against immune checkpoint proteins and novel small molecule inhibitors [49].

7. Non-Hodgkin's lymphomas (NHL)

Non-Hodgkin's lymphoma is one of the most common hematologic neoplasms and there will be an estimated in USA over 79,000 new cases and over 20,000 deaths in 2018.

Diffuse large B cell lymphoma (CD20+) is the most common type followed by follicular lymphoma and the treatment choices for patients is CHOP protocol with or without Rituximab.

7.1 Rituximab

Rituximab is achimeric anti-CD20 human monoclonal IgG1 effective directly on the surface receptor found on typical pre-B and mature B cell of non-Hodgkin's lymphoma subtypes, driving to cell cytotoxicity and cell death [53]. It was at first utilized in aggressive and very aggressive relapsed or refractory lymphoma and demonstrated safety with disease regression and free survival [54].

Major toxicities patients with NHL include infusion-related fever chills, fatigue, pruritus, nausea, and vomiting, angioedema, *headache, hypotension, bronchospasm*, urticaria during the first infusion. Rituximab was approved in November 1997 for medical use of refractory or relapsed lymphoma (B-cell). Rituximab play excellent role in combination with chemotherapy and represents a paradigm shift in treatment of lymphomas and improve the outcome for all CD20+ NHL and CLL [55].

7.2 Radioimmunotherapy

Radioimmunotherapy (RIT) is a safe and effective treatment option that combines the advantages of radiotherapy and immunotherapy and advance the adequacy of anti-CD20 target therapy by combining the antibody with a radioconjugate, yttrium-90 without risk of secondary malignancies.

7.2.1 Ibritumomab tiuxetan

Is a monoclonal antibody of IgG1 kappa with name (Zevalin) and the first radiopharmaceuticals to be approved for patients with NHL of B lymphocytes CD20 molecules. Ibritumomab linking to the metal chelator tiuxetan, a monoclonal antibody (111In Zevalin™, Biogen Idec) stable binding of indium-111 (111In) for radionucleotide tumor possible with 90Y ibritumomab tiuxetan [56].

FDA in February 2002 approved 90Y ibritumomab tiuxetan for treatment of refractory and relapsing indolent follicular lymphoma or transformed lymphoma which include lymphoma refractory to rituximab.

The toxicity of ibritumomab tiuxetan is primarily hematologic, which is both transient and reversible. The common side effects, nausea, vomiting, drug interactions, *diarrhea, cough and dizziness.*

7.2.2 Tositumomab iodine I 131

Is a CD20 radiotherapeutic targets for treatment of lymphoma patients with positive CD20 especially cases of indolent low grade lymphoma, transformed lymphoma, refractory and relapsed lymphoma and lymphoma refractory to rituximab.

The therapeutic administration protocol contain two separate products of tositumomab and iodine I131 tositumomab which will be given in two different steps include dosimetric dose and therapeutic dose separated by 10 days interval.

A relapsed, refractory, or transformed indolent low grade lymphoma overall response (OR) rates have ranged from approximately 60–80% and CR rates have ranged from about 20–40% and a median duration of response of 2 years [57].

Tositumomab toxicities include severe and prolonged thrombocytopenia and neutropenia as well as increase risk of developing other diseases include hypothyroidism, myelodysplasia, acute leukemia.

In June 2003, Tositumomab approved by FDA for treatment of CD20+ follicular lymphoma, that was relapsed following chemotherapy or lymphomas refractory to rituximab.

7.3 Denileukin diftitox

Denileukin diftitox (Ontak) is a fusion protein (interleukin 2 and diphtheria toxin) approved by FDA in October 16, 2008, for use as an antineoplastic agent to treat pretreated patients with CD25 positive cutaneous T cell lymphomas that express IL-2 receptors. A phase III clinical trial, had good response and significant improvements in self-rated overall QOL [58].

Denileukin diftitox is available in solution in 2 mL single use vials of 150 μg/mL (300 mcg in 2 mL) under the brand name Ontak. The typical dose of intravenous infusion is 9 or 18 mcg/kg/day given for 8 courses every 3 weeks.

Epratuzumab is an antihuman CD22 IgG1 antibody that targets CD22 antigen, found on the surface of B-lymphocytes antigen, CD22 [59, 60]. This drug, either in single administration or in combination with rituximab, created promising outcomes with complete remission [CR] and an ORR of 67% [49].

7.4 Ofatumumab

In August 2009, ofatumumab was approved as a high-affinity IgG1 mAb that binds to a membrane-proximal epitope of the CD20 molecule of the B cell with potential anti-neoplastic activity triggering and exhibited greater induction of complement-dependent cell lysis (CDCL) and antibody-dependent cell-mediated cytotoxicity (ADCC) of B cells over expressing CD20 when compared with rituximab [61].

7.5 Obinutuzumab

Is a unique monoclonal antibody, designed to attach to CD20 antigen expressed on the surface of pre-B- and mature B-lymphocytes of malignant lymphoma and for maintenance treatment of patients previously untreated low grade lymphoma especially follicular type resulted in significant free survival. The post-translational glycoengineering process used in the development of this agent, add to its higher binding affinity for human FcγRIII receptors on immune effector cells and the mAbs to novel targets are being developed with ADCC in mind [62].

7.6 Brentuximab vedotin

An anti-CD30 antibody-drug conjugate and demonstrated significant clinical activity in patients with CD30⁺ malignancies, including Reed Sternberg cells in classical HL and anaplastic large cell lymphoma (ALCL) (**Tables 4** and 5).

8. Multiple myeloma

Multiple myeloma (MM) is a blood cancer that remains serious disease and it cannot usually be cured because most patients relapse after treatment or become refractory to the treatments.

Novel agents are as of now in advancement for the management of refractory or relapsed multiple myeloma, counting immunomodulatory drugs, monoclonal antibodies, proteasome inhibitors, cell signaling focused on treatments, and procedures focusing on the tumor infiltration or metastasis.

Proteasome inhibitors such as bortezomib target therapy of multiple myeloma the ubiquitin pathway, coming about in cytotoxic damage due to disturbance of protein corruption in myeloma cells. The immunomodulatory agents, thalidomide, lenalidomide, and pomalidomide, are a novel of class of oral target agents impact on myeloma cells through a few components counting coordinate cytotoxicity, antiangiogenic impacts, and antitumor immunity activation (**Figure 1**).

8.1 Proteasome inhibitors

The proteasome is a gigantic highly sophisticated protease complex that degrades unneeded or damaged proteins by proteolysis. As such, the proteasome plays an important role in critical cellular processes including proliferation, differentiation, cell cycle progression and survival DNA repair, angiogenesis and apoptosis [63]. Three proteasome inhibitors, carfilzomib, bortezomib and ixazomib are approved by FDA and oprozomib and other agents are in the clinical trials late stages.

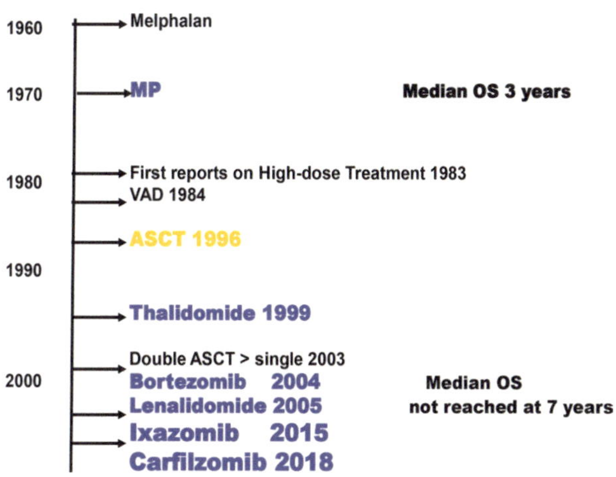

Figure 1.
History of multiple myeloma treatment.

8.2 Bortezomib

Bortezomib (Velcade) is the first proteasome inhibitor approved by FDA in May 2003. A trial phase I explored bortezomib for its tolerance and safety in multiple myeloma, lymphoma, leukemia and lung cancers [64]. Bortezomib showed safely tolerability with few side effects such as general weakness, fever, fatigue, decreased sensation and paresthesia, nausea, vomiting and thrombocytopenia. Amazing response rate (35%) and response duration reaching to more than 1 year in intensely pretreated multiple myeloma patients were reported in the SUMMIT phase II trial [65].

8.3 Carfilzomib

Carfilzomib is a new intravenous agent approved by FDA in 2018 for multiple myeloma of proteasome inhibitors like bortezomib. It should be given with dexamethasone or with dexamethasone and lenalidomide in refractory or relapsed multiple myeloma. In differentiate carfilzomib with bortezomib, appears a better selectivity to the proteasome, covering more of the proteolytic subunits. The common side effects are mild to moderate fever, cytopenia, diarrhea, headache and swelling in hands and feet [66].

8.4 Ixazomib

FDA approved ixazomib in 2015 as the first an oral proteasome inhibitor. Ixazomib used in the same time with dexamethasone and lenalidomide for the treatment patients with refractory or relapsed multiple myeloma [67].

8.5 Immunomodulatory drugs (IMiDs)

The presentation of immunomodulatory drugs (IMiDs), assist progressed long-term survival of patients with multiple myeloma. Thalidomide and its derivatives, lenalidomide and pomalidomide possess pleiotropic anti-myeloma properties including immune-modulation, anti-angiogenic, anti-inflammatory and anti-proliferative effects.

8.6 Monoclonal antibodies (MoAbs)

Presentation of the primary mAb different therapy of multiple myeloma started a modern time in multiple myeloma therapy. Daratumumab, focusing on CD38 as an exceedingly and constantly expressed surface antigen of myeloma, is the primary counter acting agent that was approved by the FDA for the treatment of newly-diagnosed multiple myeloma and also for refractory and relapsed myeloma patients [68]. Elotuzumab, targeting signaling lymphocytic activation molecule F7 (SLAMF7), has been endorsed in combination with lenalidomide and dexamethasone for therapy of myeloma patients in relapse or refractory to treatment [69].

8.7 Histone-deacetylase (HDAC) inhibitors

An assortment of epigenetic changes together with hereditary changes is basic for malignant growth and proliferation. Altering acetylation status of histones is, close by DNA methylation, an option to gene alteration and blocks gene transcription and inhibits differentiation, providing a rationale for developing HDAC inhibitors. Panobinostat was excessively attempted with different mixes in a few clinical stage I/II trials.

DOI: http://dx.doi.org/10.5772/intechopen.84696

Author details

Safa Shukry[1]*, Fadhel Hariri[2] and Abdul Wahab Al-Nehmi[3]

1 Faculty of Medicine and Health Sciences, University of Aden, Aden, Yemen

2 Supreme Authority of Medicines, Ministry of Public Health, Aden, Yemen

3 National Oncology Center, Sana'a, Yemen

*Address all correspondence to: safa_shukry@yahoo.com

References

[1] Peters S, Adjei AA. MET: A promising anticancer therapeutic target. Nature Reviews Clinical Oncology. 2012;**9**(6):314-326. DOI: 10.1038/nrclinonc.2012.71

[2] Joo WD, Visintin I, Mor G. Targeted cancer therapy—Are the days of systemic chemotherapy numbered. Maturitas. 2013;**76**(4):308-314. DOI: 10.1016/j.maturitas.2013.09.008

[3] Ross JS, Schenkein DP, Pietrusko R, et al. Targeted therapies for cancer. American Journal of Clinical Pathology. 2004;**122**:598-609. DOI: 10.1309/5CWP-U41A-FR1V-YM3F

[4] US Food and Drug Administration, Office of Combination Products. Annual Report to Congress: Federal Food, Drug, and Cosmetic Act as amended by the Medical Device User Fee Act of 2002. Rockville, MD: National Press Office; 2003

[5] Gerber DE. Targeted therapies: A new generation of cancer treatments. American Family Physician. 2008;**77**:311-319

[6] Abdul HG. Targeted therapy in oncology: A key player in the move towards personalized medicine. Journal of Developing Drugs. 2012;**1**:e116. DOI: 10.4172/2167-0714.1000e11

[7] Chauhan D, Tian Z, Nicholson B, et al. A small molecule inhibitor of ubiquitin-specific protease-7 induces apoptosis in multiple myeloma cells and overcomes bortezomib resistance. Cancer Cell. 2012;**22**(3):345-358. DOI: 10.1016/j.ccr.2012.08.007

[8] Cheson BD, Leonard JP, et al. Monoclonal antibody therapy for B-cell non-Hodgkin's lymphoma. The New England Journal of Medicine. 2008;**359**:613-626. DOI: 10.1056/NEJMra0708875

[9] Richardson PG, Weller E, Lonial S. Lenalidomide, bortezomib, and dexamethasone combination therapy in patients with newly diagnosed multiple myeloma. Blood. 2010;**116**(5):679-686. DOI: 10.1182/blood-2010-02-268862. Epub 2010 Apr 12

[10] Pittman J, Huang E, Dressman H, et al. Integrated modeling of clinical and gene expression information for personalized prediction of disease outcomes. Proceedings of the National Academy of Sciences of the United States of America. 2004;**101**:8431-8436. DOI: 10.1073/pnas.0401736101

[11] Tallman MS, Andersen JW, Schiffer CA, et al. All-trans retinoic acid in acute promyelocytic leukemia: Long-term outcome and prognostic factor analysis from north American intergroup protocol. Blood. 2002;**100**:4298-4302. DOI: 10.1182/blood-2002-02-0632. Epub 2002 Aug 15

[12] Sanz MA, Martin G, Gonzalez M, et al. Risk-adapted treatment of acute promyelocytic leukemia with all-trans-retinoic acid and anthracycline monochemotherapy: A multicenter study by the PETHEMA group. Blood. 2004;**103**:1237-1243. DOI: 10.1182/blood-2003-07-2462

[13] Estey EH, Garcia-Manero G, Ferrajoli A. Use of all-transretinoic acid (ATRA) + arsenic trioxide (ATO) to eliminate or minimize use of chemotherapy (CT) in untreated acute promyelocytic leukemia (APL). Blood. 2006;**107**(9):3469-3473. DOI: 10.1182/blood-2005-10-4006

[14] Nabhan C, Tallman MS. Early phase I/II trilas with gemtuzumab ozogamicin (Mylotarg) in acute myeloid leukemia. Clinical Lymphoma. 2002;**2**(Suppl 1):S19-S23

[15] Bross PF, Beitz J, Chen G, et al. Approval summary: Gemtuzumab

ozogamicin in relapsed acute myeloid leukemia. Clinical Cancer Research. 2001;**7**:1490-1496

[16] Sievers EL, Linenberger M. Mylotarg: Antibody-targeted chemotherapy comes of age. Current Opinion in Oncology. 2001;**13**:522-527

[17] Giles FJ, Kantarjian HM, Kornblau SM, et al. Mylotarg (gemtuzumab ozogamicin) therapy is associated with hepatic venoocclusive disease in patients who have not received stem cell transplantation. Cancer. 2001;**92**:406-413

[18] Shaheen RM, Davis DW, Liu W, et al. Antiangiogenic therapy targeting the tyrosine kinase receptor for vascular endothelial growth factor receptor inhibits the growth of colon cancer and liver metastasis and induces tumor and endothelial cell apoptosis. Cancer Research. 1999;**59**:5412-5416

[19] Masarova L, Kantarjian H, Garcia-Mannero G, et al. Harnessing the immune system against leukemia: Monoclonal antibodies and checkpoint strategies for AML. Advances in Experimental Medicine and Biology. 2017;**995**:73-95. DOI: 10.1007/978-3-319-53156-4_4

[20] Cho BS, Kim HJ, Konopleva M. Targeting the CXCL12/CXCR4 axis in acute myeloid leukemia: From bench to bedside. The Korean Journal of Internal Medicine. 2017;**32**(2):248-257. DOI: 10.3904/kjim.2016.244

[21] Nguyen B, Williams AB, Young DJ, et al. FLT3 activating mutations display differential sensitivity to multiple tyrosine kinase inhibitors. Oncotarget. 2017;**8**(7):10931-10944. DOI: 10.18632/oncotarget.14539

[22] Amatangelo MD, Quek L, Shih A, et al. Enasidenib induces acute myeloid leukemia cell differentiation to promote clinical response. Blood. 2017;**130**(6):732-741. DOI: 10.1182/blood-2017-04-779447

[23] Soderquist R, Eastman A. BCL2 inhibitors as anticancer drugs: A plethora of misleading BH3 mimetics. Molecular Cancer Therapeutics. 2016;**15**(9):2011-2017. DOI: 10.1158/1535-7163.MCT-16-0031

[24] Jamieson GC, Fox JA, Poi M, et al. Molecular and pharmacologic properties of the anticancer quinolone derivative vosaroxin: A new therapeutic agent for acute myeloid leukemia. Drugs. 2016;**76**(13):1245-1255. DOI: 10.1007/s40265-016-0614-z

[25] Zhao J, Xie C, Edwards H, et al. Histone deacetylases 1 and 2 cooperate in regulating BRCA1, CHK1, and RAD51 expression in acute myeloid leukemia cells. Oncotarget. 2017;**8**(4):6319-6329. DOI: 10.18632/oncotarget.14062

[26] Montalban-Bravo G, Huang X, Jabbour E, et al. A clinical trial for patients with acute myeloid leukemia or myelodysplastic syndromes not eligible for standard clinical trials. Leukemia. 2017;**31**(2):318-324. DOI: 10.1038/leu.2016.303

[27] Lee KH, Choi SJ, Lee JH. Imatinib plus combination chemotherapy for newly-diagnosed Philadelphia chromosome-positive acute lymphoblastic leukemia. Blood. 2003;**102**:884a. Abstract 3288

[28] Thomas DA, Cortes J, Giles FJ, et al. Rituximab and hyper-CVAD for adult Burkitt's (BL) or Burkitt's like (BL) leukemia or lymphoma. Blood. 2002;**100**:763a

[29] Ozsahin H, Fluss J, McLin V, et al. Rituximab with interleukin-2 after autologous bone marrow transplantation for acute lymphocytic leukemia in second remission. Medical and Pediatric Oncology. 2002;**38**:300-301

[30] Kantarjian H, Ravandi F, Short NJ, et al. Inotuzumab ozogamicin in combination with low-intensity chemotherapy for older patients with Philadelphia chromosome-negative acute lymphoblastic leukaemia: A single-arm, phase 2 study. The Lancet Oncology. 2018;**19**(2):240-248. DOI: 10.1016/S1470-2045(18)30011-1. Epub 2018 Jan 16

[31] Kantarjian H, Stein A, Gökbuget N, et al. Blinatumomab versus chemotherapy for advanced acute lymphoblastic leukemia. The New England Journal of Medicine. 2017;**376**:836-847. DOI: 10.1056/NEJMoa1609783

[32] Lew G, Gu L, Zhou M, et al. BL22, an anti-CD22 recombinant immunotoxin, is active in vitro and in vivo against B-cell precursor acute lymphoblastic leukemia (BCP-ALL) cells from pediatric patients. Blood. 2002;**100**:764a. Abstract 3024

[33] Kolitz JE, Omara V, Willemze R, et al. Treatment of acute lymphoblastic leukemia with campath-1H: Initial observations. Blood. 1994;**84**:301a. Abstract 1191

[34] Abdul Hamid G. Target therapy and monitoring of chronic myeloid leukemia. World Journal of Pharmaceutical Research. 2015;**4**(9):391-405

[35] Kantarjian HM, Dixon D, Keating MJ, et al. Characteristics of accelerated disease in chronic myelogenous leukemia. Cancer. 1988;**61**:1441

[36] Abdul-Rahman SA, Hamid GA, Nasher S, et al. Chronic myeloid leukemia in South Yemen. International Journal of Biopharmaceutical Sciences. 2018;**1**(2):110. DOI: 10.31021/ijbs.20181110

[37] Goldman JM, Melo JV. Targeting the BCR-ABL tyrosine kinase in chronic myeloid leukemia. The New England Journal of Medicine. 2001;**344**:1084-1086

[38] Jabbour E, Cortes JE, Kantarjian HM. Suboptimal response to or failure of imatinib treatment for chronic myeloid leukemia: What is the optimal strategy? Mayo Clinic Proceedings. 2009;**84**:161-169. PMC2664587

[39] Talpaz M, Shah NP, Kantarjian H, et al. Dasatinib in imatinib-resistant Philadelphia chromosome-positive leukemias. The New England Journal of Medicine. 2006;**354**:2531-2541. DOI: 10.1056/NEJMoa055229

[40] Kantarjian H, Shah N, Hochhaus A, et al. Dasatinib versus imatinib in newly diagnosed chronic-phase chronic myeloid leukemia. The New England Journal of Medicine. 2010;**362**(24):2260-2270. DOI: 10.1056/NEJMoa1002315. Epub 2010 Jun 5

[41] Saglio G, Dong-Wook K, Issaragrisill S, et al. Nilotinib versus imatinib for newly diagnosed chronic myeloid leukemia. The New England Journal of Medicine. 2010;**362**(24):2251-2259. DOI: 10.1056/NEJMoa0912614

[42] Khoury HJ, Cortes JE, Kantarjian HE, et al. Bosutinib is active in chronic phase chronic myeloid leukemia after imatinib and dasatinib and/or nilotinib therapy failure. Blood. 2012;**119**(15):3403-3412. DOI: 10.1182/blood-2011-11-390120

[43] Verma D, Kantarjian HM, Jones D, et al. Chronic myeloid leukemia (CML) with P190 BCR-ABL: Analysis of characteristics, outcomes, and prognostic significance. Blood. 2009;**114**(11):2232-2235. DOI: 10.1182/blood-2009-02-204693

[44] Marin D, Milojkovic D, Olavarria E, et al. European LeukemiaNet criteria for failure or sub-optimal response reliably identify patients with CML in early

chronic phase treated with imatinib whose eventual outcome is poor. Blood. 2008;**112**:4437-4444. DOI: 10.1182/blood-2008-06-162388

[45] Gouri A, Dekaken A, Chefrour M, et al. Molecular monitoring of chronic myeloid leukemia (CML): A current perspective. Journal of Hematology and Thromboembolic Diseases. 2015;**3**:2. DOI: 10.4172/2329-8790.1000e118

[46] Baccarani M, Cortes J, Pane F, et al. European LeukemiaNet. Chronic myeloid leukemia: An update of concepts and management recommendations of European LeukemiaNet. Journal of Clinical Oncology. 2009;**27**(35):6041-6051

[47] Molica S. Sex difference in incidence and outcome of chronic lymphocytic leukemia patients. Leukemia & Lymphoma. 2006;**47**:1477-1480. DOI: 10.1080/10428190600555819

[48] Hendriks RW, Yuvaraj S, Kil LP. Targeting Bruton's tyrosine kinase in B cell malignancies. Nature Reviews. Cancer. 2014;**14**(4):219-223. DOI: 10.1038/nrc3702

[49] Grover NS, Park SI. Novel targeted agents in Hodgkin's and non-Hodgkin's lymphoma therapy. Pharmaceutical. 2015;**8**:607-636. DOI: 10.3390/ph8030607

[50] Furman RR, Sharman JP, Steven E, et al. Idelalisib and rituximab in relapsed chronic lymphocytic leukemia. The New England Journal of Medicine. 2014;**370**:997-1007. DOI: 10.1056/NEJMoa1315226

[51] Nabhan C, Rosen ST. Chronic lymphocytic leukemia: A clinical review. Journal of the American Medical Association. 2014;**312**(21):2265-2276. DOI: 10.1001/jama.2014.14553

[52] Roberts AW, Davids MS, Pagel JM, et al. Targeting BCL2 with venetoclax in relapsed chronic lymphocytic leukemia. The New England Journal of Medicine. 2016;**374**:311-322. DOI: 10.1056/NEJMoa1513257

[53] Bello C, Sotomayor EM. Monoclonal antibodies for B-cell lymphomas: Rituximab and beyond. In: Hematology ASH Education Program. 2007;**2007**:233-242. PMID: 18024635. Available from: http://dx.doi.org/10.1182/asheducation-2007.1.233

[54] Grillo-Lopez AJ, Hedrick E, Rashford M, et al. Rituximab: Ongoing and future clinical development. Seminars in Oncology. 2002;**29** (1 Suppl. 2):105-112

[55] Coiffier B, Lepage E, Briere J, et al. CHOP chemotherapy plus rituximab compared with CHOP alone in elderly patients with diffuse large-B-cell lymphoma. The New England Journal of Medicine. 2002;**346**:235-242. DOI: 10.1056/NEJMoa011795

[56] Wagner HN Jr, Wiseman GA, Marcus CS, et al. Administration guidelines for radioimmunotherapy of non-Hodgkin's lymphoma with 90Y-labeled anti CD20 monoclonal antibody. Journal of Nuclear Medicine. 2002;**43**:267-272

[57] Kaminski MS, Zelenetz AD, Press OW, et al. Pivotal study of iodine I131 tositumomab for chemotherapy-refractory low-grade or transformed low grade B-cell non-Hodgkin's lymphomas. Journal of Clinical Oncology. 2001;**19**:3918-3928

[58] Olsen E, Duvic M, Frankel A, et al. Pivotal phase III trial of two dose levels of denileukin diftitox for the treatment of cutaneous T-cell lymphoma. Journal of Clinical Oncology. 2001;**19**:376-388

[59] Shih LB, Lu HH, Xuan H, et al. Internalization and intracellular processing of anti-B-cell lymphoma

monoclonal antibody, LL2. International Journal of Cancer. 1994;**56**:538-545

[60] Gada P, Hernandez-Ilizalituri FJ, Repasky EA, et al. Epratuzumab's predominant anti-tumor activity in vitro/in vivo against non-Hodgkin's lymphoma (NHL) is via antibody-dependent cellular cytotoxicity (ADCC). Blood. 2002;**100**:1367a

[61] Karlin L, Coiffier B. Ofatumumab in the treatment of non-Hodgkin's lymphomas. Expert Opinion on Biological Therapy. 2015;**15**(7):1085-1091. DOI: 10.1517/14712598.2015.1055241. Epub 2015 Jun 4

[62] Marcus R, Davies A, Ando K, et al. Obinutuzumab for the first-line treatment of follicular lymphoma. The New England Journal of Medicine. 2017;**377**:1331-1344. DOI: 10.1056/NEJMoa1614598

[63] Schmidt M, Finley D. Regulation of proteasome activity in health and disease. Biochimica et Biophysica Acta. 2014;**1843**:13-25. DOI: 10.1016/j.bbamcr.2013.08.012

[64] Orlowski RZ, Stinchcombe TE, Mitchell BS, et al. Phase I trial of the proteasome inhibitor PS-341 in patients with refractory hematologic malignancies. Journal of Clinical Oncology. 2002;**20**:4420-4427. DOI: 10.1200/JCO.2002.01.133

[65] Richardson PG, Barlogie B, Berenson J, et al. A phase 2 study of bortezomib in relapsed, refractory myeloma. The New England Journal of Medicine. 2003;**348**:2609-2617. DOI: 10.1056/NEJMoa030288

[66] Shah C, Bishnoi R, Wang Y, et al. Efficacy and safety of carfilzomib in relapsed and/o refractory multiple myeloma: Systematic review and meta-analysis of 14 trials. Oncotarget. 2018;**9**:23704-23717. DOI: 10.18632/oncotarget.25281

[67] Richardson PG, Baz R, Wang M, et al. Phase 1 study of twice-weekly ixazomib, an oral proteasome inhibitor in relapsed/refractory multiple myeloma patients. Blood. 2014;**124**:1038-1046. DOI: 10.1182/blood-2014-01-548826

[68] Mateos MV, Dimopoulos MA, Cavo M, et al. Daratumumab plus Bortezomib, Melphalan, and prednisone for untreated myeloma. The New England Journal of Medicine. 2018;**378**:518-528. DOI: 10.1056/NEJMoa1714678

[69] Lonial S, Dimopoulos M, Palumbo A, et al. Elotuzumab therapy for relapsed or refractory multiple myeloma. The New England Journal of Medicine. 2015;**373**:621-631. DOI: 10.1056/NEJMoa1505654

Chapter 8

Perceptions and Challenges for Adoption of Generics and Biosimilars in Oncology

Amit Garg, Deepak CSN and Tarveen Jandoo

Abstract

Cancer care is increasingly becoming challenging in low resource settings. With the improved availability and access of generic medicines and biosimilars, cost-effective and affordable treatment can be offered to cancer patients. However, generics and biosimilars continue to be plagued with negative perceptions that impact the adoption of these products. Lack of understanding and negative perceptions regarding the quality, safety, effectiveness, integrity and stability, formulations, manufacturing, and costs of generics and biosimilars are more common in the developing countries. Their equivalence to innovator counterparts is often doubted. Collaborative efforts for enhanced utilization of generics and biosimilars in oncology should be made by physicians, healthcare professionals, manufacturers and sponsors of these drugs, and national healthcare systems. Steps to improve access and utilization of these drugs include procurement of high-quality generics and biosimilars, formulary management, supply chain integrity, continued safety surveillance, and educational programs to improve knowledge mitigate fears in healthcare professionals and patients. Objective and standard frameworks should be developed and used to identify the perceptions and factors impacting the adoption of generics and biosimilars. Outcomes in hematological malignancies can be improved with the adoption of generics and biosimilars, in particular in low-income countries where access and affordability of chemotherapy is challenging.

Keywords: generics, biosimilars, perceptions, adoption, oncology

1. Introduction

Generic medicines find application in both chemotherapy and supportive care in oncology. Generics are increasingly available for small molecules and biologic agents used in oncology treatment regimens.

Generic medicines are pharmaceutical drugs that have the same chemical substance, i.e., the same active pharmaceutical ingredient (API), as that of the originator drug. According to the US Food and Drug Administration (FDA), "a generic drug is a medication created to be the same as an existing approved brand-name drug in dosage form, safety, strength, route of administration, quality, performance characteristics, and intended use [1]." According to the European Medicines Agency (EMA), "a generic medicine is developed to be the same as a medicine that has already been authorized, called the reference

Parameter	Generic drug	Biosimilar
Manufacturing	Simple and predictable	Stepwise to produce compound as similar as possible to the originator biologic
Immunogenicity	Low potential	No increase in comparison to the reference biologic
Regulatory approvals	Small trials in healthy volunteers/patients	At least one study including assessments of pharmacokinetics, pharmacodynamics, and immunogenicity

Table 1.
Key differences between generic medicines and biosimilar agents.

medicine [2]." These regulatory directions of similarity imply the possible substitution of innovator products with generic medicines. According to the World Health Organization (WHO), a generic is a 'multisource pharmaceutical product which is intended to be interchangeable with the comparator product.' This also includes an originator brand for which the patent has expired. WHO has distinguished between originator brand, regardless of its patent status, and lowest-priced generic equivalents [3]. Biosimilars are defined as biologic products that are highly similar to reference products, notwithstanding minor differences in clinically inactive components. Biosimilars have no clinically meaningful differences to the reference product in terms of safety profile, purity, and potency [4]. Both generics and biosimilars are widely used in cancer care. However, there are several differences between the two agents (**Table 1**) [5].

Generic medicines may differ from the originator products in the manufacturing processes. There may be subtle differences in the excipients, color, and packaging. Sometimes, generic medicines may also have different formulations. According to the EMA, "a generic medicine's inactive ingredients, name, appearance and packaging can be different [2]." Approval of generics and biosimilars are granted after confirmation of evidence of biophysical similarity to the originator reference products. This is a proxy to similarity in the clinical effectiveness and safety of generics and biosimilars. Generics and biosimilars are approved only when there is 'totality of evidence' for similarity to the reference originator product. This includes robust scientific data for parameters of structural analysis, preclinical, pharmacokinetic, efficacy and safety, and immunogenicity.

2. Regulations around generics

Various countries have regulations for the development and availability of generic medicines. Generic medicines can be marked in a country only after a marketing authorization has been obtained. The US FDA requires generics to be identical to the originator products in pharmacokinetic and pharmacodynamic properties. There are defined parameters for establishment of bioequivalence of generic medicines to their branded counterparts. The FDA's Office of Generic Drugs (OGD) has a vigorous review process facilitating the approval of generic medicines of high quality [6]. The FDA also has clear directions for the development, review, and approval of biosimilars [7]. In the EU, the EMA reviews the quality standards and other parameters to establish the equivalence of a generic medicine to its innovator counterpart [8]. Various countries have described regulations for the production, review, and approval of generics though the regulatory frameworks are not equally mature in all countries [9, 10].

3. Use and impact of generics

Generic medicines are increasingly being used in most countries across the world. In the US, 9 out of 10 prescriptions are said to have a generic drug [1]. In the European Union (EU), about 20–80% prescriptions are filled with generics [11]. However, lower utilization of generics is reported in the lesser developed countries [12]. Not all generic medicines are available in all countries. Both generics and biosimilars are widely used in hematological malignancies. Examples include lenalidomide for multiple myeloma, rituximab for Non-Hodgkin's lymphoma, chronic lymphocytic leukemia, and filgrastim for febrile neutropenia.

3.1 Cost reduction

Generic medicines are lesser priced when compared to the innovator products and offer affordable options in management of various disease conditions including cancer [4, 13]. This has special relevance in low-income countries as it improves access and compliance to therapeutic options. Treatment regimens are associated with huge costs in oncology settings. The lesser price of generics and biosimilars is reflective of the abbreviated pathways to regulatory approvals.

The widespread use of generics has favorably influenced the national healthcare spending. The utilization of generics is influenced by various factors such as physician recommendations, pharmacy practices, patient preferences, and the economic status of the patient. The use of biosimilars is reported to have an average of 20–30% cost-saving effect [14].

3.2 Improved compliance

The affordability of generics and biosimilars offers an opportunity for sustained engagement and adherence of patients to the treatment regimens [15]. This is of greater relevance in oncology where therapeutic options are expensive and treatments last long periods [16]. High costs of treatment are a common impediment in the management of cancer. Reduction of costs leads to enhanced access and adoption of generics [17, 18].

4. Perceptions and adoption of generics

Though generic medicines have been available for several decades, there is paucity of knowledge about what these medicines are and how these differ from their innovator counterparts. There is also a lack of understanding about the standards described for the approval and market authorization of generics and how these drugs have a lower cost [19].

There are lacunae in knowledge about generics in physicians, healthcare professionals, and patients. This is evident in the perceptions that healthcare professionals and patients have for generics and biosimilars. These perceptions drive the apathy or antipathy for generics and impact the adoption of generics in routine practice. There are mixed perceptions regarding the use of generic medicines. The perceptions differ in various countries. While physicians in the high-income countries generally have positive perceptions for generics, those in the low-income countries generally have more negative perceptions [12, 20]. Controversies have emerged regarding the adoption of generics for brand substitution [21]. The differences in perceptions can be attributed to various factors including the regulatory milieu, healthcare policies, educational initiatives, and drug information sources.

Perceptions regarding generics and biosimilars and attitudes of physicians, healthcare providers, and patients impact the use of generics (**Figure 1**). Several factors may impact the acceptance and use of generics. These factors are diverse and include increased knowledge about the regulated approval of generics and biosimilars and the increased awareness regarding generics from the access to information in social and scientific platforms.

Perceptions and levers for adoption of generics may be grouped into four broad categories (**Figure 2**).

4.1 Effectiveness

Though generic medicines have an established equal effectiveness to their innovator counterparts and are intended to be interchangeable with the latter, they

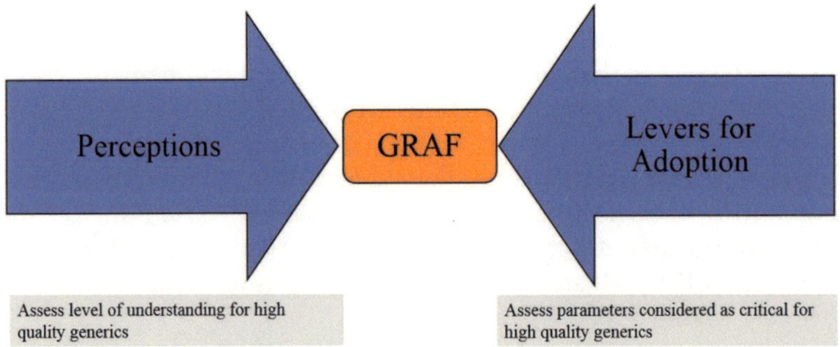

Figure 1.
Use and adoption of generics and biosimilars. GRAF (generic dRug adoption framework) is a tool to identify and differentiate high quality generics.

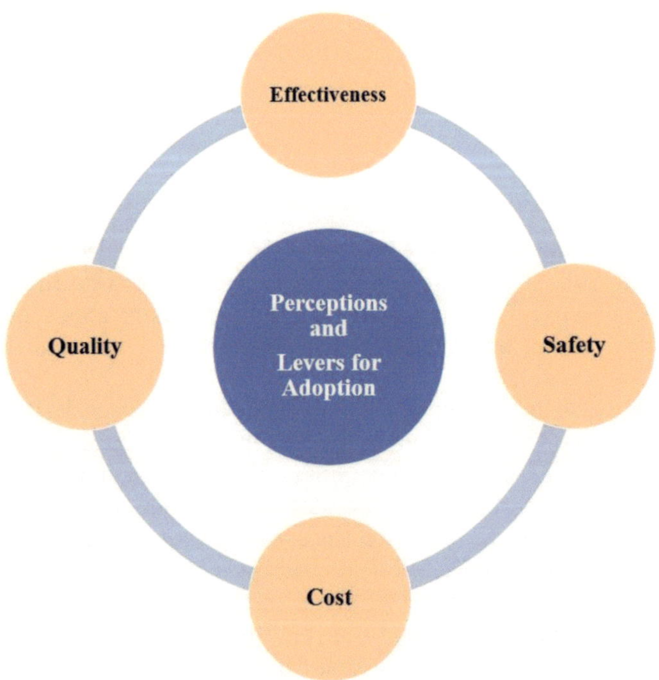

Figure 2.
Components of perceptions and levers for adoption of generics.

are perceived to be less efficacious effective. Physicians and healthcare professionals need to understand how confirmation of similar clinical outcomes is key to the regulatory review process for the approval of generics and biosimilars. Bioequivalence is a standard and reliable measure to confirm the similar effectiveness of generics and their branded counterparts. Bioequivalence is a dependable proxy for similar clinical effects [22]. Therapeutic benefits are maintained when patients receiving innovator drugs are switched over to generic options of the same dosing. In the setting of oncology, this switch is not reported to impact the cytogenetic or molecular response [23]. The demonstration of equivalence and increasing awareness for the same can help physicians and healthcare professionals in easy decision making for a switch to generic options.

4.2 Safety

The likely differences in manufacturing and excipients between generics and innovator products raise concerns about the safety of generics. Safety is usually measured in terms of the number and frequency of adverse effects with the clinical use of a pharmaceutical product. There is no established evidence for the inferiority of generic medicines for any safety parameters. However, there is a growing trend towards the enhanced reporting of safety experiences with generics. This is suggestive of increased surveillance for the safety of generics [24, 25].

Continued safety monitoring is increasingly being applied to generics and biosimilars. Any efforts made to set up such systems build trust and acceptance for the generic molecules. The exposure of generics to stringent pharmacovigilance practices in the regulated markets are a proxy to established safety of the products. The safety monitoring systems in the regulated markets are mature and reliable. These systems allow for the easy identification of generics in the reports. For example, in the US, the FDA adverse event reporting system (FEARS) enables the identification of generic drugs in the safety reporting systems [26]. If approved and marketed in countries with such regulations, generic medicines are perceived to hold a promise of safety. This facilitates the easy adoption of such approved products.

4.3 Cost

Generic medicines and biosimilars are perceived as low-cost alternatives to expensive originator anticancer drugs. Many patients perceive generics as less efficacious; physicians and pharmacists continue to doubt the safety of generics [27]. These perceptions impact the utilization of generics.

There are smaller price differentials between biosimilars and biopharmaceuticals when compared to generics and their comparator originators. This is explained by the longer development time and larger research costs for biosimilars. Cost-effectiveness and cost-utility analyses are being used to establish the economic benefits of adopting biosimilars. Such economic evaluations have a role in checking the rapidly rising healthcare expenditures [28]. However, there is a lack of regulatory directions for the most appropriate techniques of economic evaluation for generics and biosimilars.

The benefits of cost saving options are manifold. Patients may seek affordable options, physicians may be reassured by the willingness and ability of patients to complete the therapy, and payers may view this as a pharmacoeconomic reform. The WHO has described cost of therapy as a key component of rational prescribing [29].

Payers, physicians, and patients are developing an incline to evaluate the pharmacoeconomics of generics and biosimilars periodically throughout the life cycle of the product. This is explained by the increasingly available experience in the real-world settings with these products. Economic efficiency is not solely determined by the relative costs of generics and comparators. It is ideally defined by the attainable levels of efficiency and safety with the use of lower-priced options. This eventually constitutes the quality of the generics and biosimilars [30]. In a cost minimization study in Colombia, use of generic equivalents of bortezomib, decitabine and capecitabine resulted in substantial savings of 63% (USD 4.68 million), 26% (USD 0.29 million), and 46% (USD 1.50 million), respectively [31].

4.4 Quality

Quality is a key parameter that impacts the utilization of generics. It is important to understand the perceptions about quality of generics and also define what parameters define quality of generics.

The regulatory standards for approval of generics and biosimilars are guided by the principles of quality by design (QbD) [32]. This implies that science-driven and risk-based concepts underlie the development, scale-up, and manufacturing of generics and biosimilars. The yield of this approach is a high-quality generic product or biosimilar molecule with an implied clinical equivalence which may be validated in research studies and clinical experience. Quality is not alone limited to structural and chemical similarities during development; it also spans to the similarities of generic drugs to comparators in final formulations and packaging. Quality is also defined by testing for stability, sterility, and impurities. These data are an important and mandatory component of abbreviated new drug applications (ANDAs) [33]. The WHO has defined standards for good manufacturing practices (GMP) as a guide to the quality assurance of pharmaceutical products [34].

5. Challenges for switch and adoption

With the prevalent perceptions about generics, there are several likely challenges that physicians and patients can confront for the adoption of these drugs. Observational studies have confirmed doubts and unfavorable attitudes in physicians, pharmacists, and lay people for the effectiveness, safety, and quality of generic medicines [27]. There may be questions regarding the dependable and acceptable evidence for the effectiveness and safety of generics and biosimilars. There may be uncertainties regarding the acceptance of bioequivalence as a marker of similarity. These uncertainties may lead to cohesive discussions in media and scientific platforms which in turn may influence the decision-making for switch and substitution with generics and biosimilars.

Physicians may want to go for facility visits to understand and inspect the development and manufacturing of generics. This can build trust in the products and facilitate their early and easy adoption. Consistent product supply may be taken as a proxy to dependable quality and this can safeguard the trust in the product of a particular supplier. On the other hand, physicians may feel reassured regarding safety if the generic or biosimilar has been approved in a regulated market with clear guidance for development and approval of these products.

6. Efforts by companies and physicians

Physicians should make sustained efforts to discuss the most cost-effective therapeutic options with patients and help them to achieve desired outcomes at lower costs [35, 36]. This may be an important aspect of therapy in low income countries with majority of patients belonging to the poorer segments [37]. Many of these countries have ill-defined reimbursement policies and healthcare management is largely an out-of-pocket expense. Not alone physicians, pharmacists have an important role in the switch and substitution of generics and biosimilars [14].

Company sponsored patient assistance programs (PAP) have a huge potential to improve access to generics and biosimilars. These programs offer medicines to eligible patients at no or minimal costs [38]. Companies should also make efforts to educate patients, inform physicians, and demonstrate benefits to payers for their products.

7. Role of healthcare systems

Healthcare systems should prepare for increased adoption of generics and biosimilars by procurement and formulary management, continued safety surveillance, and transformational reforms for mitigating the economic and operational challenges. A healthcare system should aim to allow an equitable access to essential medicines of assured quality, efficacy, and safety [39]. Policies and programs should aim to not only improve access but also build trust in medicine quality and healthcare systems [40].

Procurement of high-quality generics is the first and key step that acts as a gatekeeper to the access and adoption of generics and biosimilars in a particular country. These practices need to be standardized and implemented as nation-wide initiatives for successful utilization of generics. Efforts should be made to develop and design a prequalification scheme to assist countries lacking strong regulations in procurement of anticancer generics and biosimilars of assured quality [13].

Regulators are making constant efforts to improve the knowledge and understanding for the development and clinical use of biosimilars. In collaboration with the European Commission, the EMA has formulated an information guide for healthcare professionals to educate them about the development, approval, effectiveness, safety, switch, substitution, and interchangeability of biosimilars [8]. Such efforts need to be replicated by the healthcare systems in countries with poor regulations. Manufacturers can collaborate with the healthcare systems to plan and implement educational programs for physicians, pharmacists, and patients. Physicians should be educated for the criteria of equivalence, safety and vigilance, and manufacturing processes adopted for developing high-quality generics and biosimilars.

There is lack of unawareness for the costs of pharmaceutical therapies in physicians [41]. Educational programs should aim to improve understanding for the lower costs of generics and biosimilars and the implications of this on overall cost of therapy.

Payers should be encouraged to develop appropriate reimbursement policies that will encourage the use of generic medicines in routine clinical practice. Further, a pool of generic suppliers should be identified to ensure an uninterrupted availability of these medicines [13]. Generic medicines and biosimilars should be included in the national lists of essential medicines and should be part of national formularies. The integrity of supply chains should be maintained and circulation of counterfeit or substandard products should be discouraged. Lack of constant drug supplies can lead to mistrust in patients and lack of confidence in physicians and healthcare systems. All these factors compromise clinical care in oncology where treatments are phased and last longer.

8. Recommendations

Most experience about the knowledge and perceptions regarding generics comes from interviews and surveys conducted in cross sections of populations in various countries [12, 27, 42, 43]. There is lack of a standard approach for the assessment of knowledge, attitudes, and perceptions about generics. In addition, factors impacting the utilization of generics have not been precisely determined. Sustained and collaborative efforts should be made to understand the perceptions for generic medicines and mitigate the same.

Educational initiatives should be introduced by manufacturers of generics and biosimilars and healthcare systems to improve knowledge about these drugs and develop positive attitudes towards their adoption. This will empower physicians, patients, and pharmacists to make rational choices in therapy and improve outcomes of cancer care.

Uniform standards should be developed for high-quality generics and these need to be implemented at global levels. Maiden efforts in this direction include tools like the generic dRug adoption framework (GRAF) (**Figure 1**). This framework, comprising a 20-item questionnaire, has been developed to enable physicians and pharmacists to make decisions to identify and differentiate high quality generics and facilitate interchangeability. Currently available in three languages (English, Spanish, and Portuguese), the framework has successfully been implemented in Brazil and Colombia. More and more countries should adopt such objective measures to evaluate the perceptions and adoption of high-quality generics. Insights gained from the experience of such frameworks can help to make further reforms to allow the identification, procurement, and prescription of high-quality generic medicines. This can advance the use of cost-effective solutions in cancer care.

9. Conclusions

Availability of generics and easier access to these drugs can impact the outcomes in oncology settings. The low-priced and affordable generic medicines and biosimilars can improve the adoption and compliance with treatment options in cancer care. However, the low price of these drugs is often construed as compromise in quality. There are myriad perceptions for the use of generics and biosimilars in routine practice. The perceptions are different among physicians in high- and low-income countries; these can possibly be due to differences in regulations and policies, educational opportunities and available drug information sources. Factors like cost, quality, effectiveness, and safety impact the understanding for and adoption of generics and biosimilars. There are several challenges in the substitution and switch from originator products to generics and biosimilars. The widespread and confident adoption of generics requires collaborative efforts of prescribers, healthcare professionals, payers, and the manufacturers of these agents.

Conflict of interest

The authors have no conflicts of interest.

Author details

Amit Garg[1]*, Deepak CSN[1] and Tarveen Jandoo[2]

1 Dr. Reddy's Laboratories Ltd., Hyderabad, India

2 Independent Medical Affairs Consultant, New Delhi, India

*Address all correspondence to: amitgarg@drreddys.com

References

[1] Generic Drugs. Overview & Basics. FDA. 2017. Available from: https://www.fda.gov/Drugs/ResourcesForYou/Consumers/BuyingUsingMedicineSafely/GenericDrugs/ucm567297.htm [Accessed: 25 January 2019]

[2] Generic and hybrid medicines. European Medicines Agency. Available from: https://www.ema.europa.eu/en/human-regulatory/marketing-authorisation/generic-hybrid-medicines [Accessed: 25 January 2019]

[3] Marketing Authorization of Pharmaceutical Products with Special Reference to Multisource (Generic) Products: A Manual for Drug Regulatory Authorities—Regulatory Support Series No. 005. WHO. Available from: http://apps.who.int/medicinedocs/en/d/Js2273e/ [Accessed: 31 January 2019]

[4] Ahmed I, Kaspar B, Sharma U. Biosimilars: Impact of biologic product life cycle and European experience on the regulatory trajectory in the United States. Clinical Therapeutics. 2012;**34**(2):400-419. DOI: 10.1016/j.clinthera.2011.12.005

[5] Nabhan C, Parsad S, Mato AR, Feinberg BA. Biosimilars in oncology in the United States: A review. JAMA Oncology. 2018;**4**(2):241-247. DOI: 10.1001/jamaoncol.2017.2004

[6] Approved products with therapeutic equivalence evaluations. 38th ed. Food and Drug Administration US Department of Health and Human Services. Office of Medicinal Products and Tobacco, Center for Drug Evaluation and Research, Office of Generic Drugs, Office of Generic Drug Policy; 2018. Available from: https://www.fda.gov/downloads/Drugs/DevelopmentApprovalProcess/UCM071436.pdf [Accessed: 25 January 2019]

[7] Biosimilar Development, Review, and approval. US Food and Drug Administration. Available from: https://www.fda.gov/Drugs/DevelopmentApprovalProcess/HowDrugsareDevelopedandApproved/ApprovalApplications/TherapeuticBiologicApplications/Biosimilars/ucm580429.htm [Accessed: 26 January 2019]

[8] Biosimilars in the EU. European Medicines Agency. Available from: https://www.ema.europa.eu/documents/leaflet/biosimilars-eu-information-guide-healthcare-professionals_en.pdf [Accessed: 26 January 2019]

[9] Kuribayashi R, Sawanobori K. Current Japanese regulatory systems for generics and biosimilars. Journal of Pharmaceutical Sciences. 2018;**107**(3):785-787. DOI: 10.1016/j.xphs.2017.10.040

[10] Alfonso-Cristancho R, Andia T, Barbosa T, Watanabe JH. Definition and classification of generic drugs across the world. Applied Health Economics and Health Policy. 2015;**13**(Suppl 1):S5-S11. DOI: 10.1007/s40258-014-0146-1

[11] Wouters OJ, Kanavos PG, McKEE M. Comparing generic drug markets in Europe and the United States: Prices, volumes, and spending. The Milbank Quarterly. 2017;**95**(3):554-601. DOI: 10.1111/1468-0009.12279

[12] Gebresillassie BM, Belachew SA, Tefera YG, Abebe TB, Mekuria AB, Haile KT, et al. Evaluating patients', physicians' and pharmacy professionals' perception and concern regarding generic medicines in Gondar town, Northwest Ethiopia: A multi-stakeholder, cross-sectional survey. PLoS ONE. 2018;**13**(11):e0204146. DOI: 10.1371/journal.pone.0204146. eCollection 2018

[13] Renner L, Nkansah FA, Dodoo AN. The role of generic medicines and biosimilars in oncology in low-income countries. Annals of Oncology. 2013;**24**(Suppl 5):v29-v32. DOI: 10.1093/annonc/mdt326

[14] Lucio SD, Stevenson JG, Hoffman JM. Biosimilars: Implications for health-system pharmacists. American Journal of Health-System Pharmacy. 2013;**70**(22):2004-2017. DOI: 10.2146/ajhp130119

[15] Stein JD, Shekhawat N, Talwar N, Balkrishnan R. Impact of the introduction of generic latanoprost on glaucoma medication adherence. Ophthalmology. 2015;**122940**:738-747. DOI: 10.1016/j.ophtha.2014.11.022

[16] Neuner JM, Kamaraju S, Charlson JA, Wozniak EM, Smith EC, Biggers A, et al. The introduction of generic aromatase inhibitors and treatment adherence among Medicare D enrollees. Journal of the National Cancer Institute. 2015;**107**(8):djv130. DOI: 10.1093/jnci/djv130

[17] Neugut AI, Subar M, Wilde ET, Stratton S, Brouse CH, Hillyer GC, et al. Association between prescription co-payment amount and compliance with adjuvant hormonal therapy in women with early-stage breast cancer. Journal of Clinical Oncology. 2011;**29**(18):2534-2542. DOI: 10.1200/JCO.2010.33.3179

[18] Riley GF, Warren JL, Harlan LC, Blackwell SA. Endocrine therapy use among elderly hormone receptor-positive breast cancer patients enrolled in Medicare part D. Medicare & Medicaid Research Review. 2011;**1**(4):E1-E26. DOI: 10.5600/mmrr.001.04.a04

[19] Euen BJ, Fadda HM. Community pharmacists' understanding and perceptions of FDA therapeutic equivalence standards. Research in Social & Administrative Pharmacy. 2018. pii: S1551-7411(17)30634-4. DOI: 10.1016/j.sapharm.2018.03.005

[20] Hassali MA, Wong ZY, Alrasheedy AA, Saleem F, Mohamad Yahaya AH, Aljadhey H. Perspectives of physicians practicing in low and middle income countries towards generic medicines: A narrative review. Health Policy. 2014;**117**(3):297-310. DOI: 10.1016/j.healthpol.2014.07.014

[21] Ferner RE, Lenney W, Marriott JF. Controversy over generic substitution. British Medical Journal. 2010;**340**(c2548). DOI: 10.1136/bmj.c2548

[22] Kesselheim AS, Misono AS, Lee JL, Stedman MR, Brookhart MA, Choudhry NK, et al. Clinical equivalence of generic and brand-name Drugs used in cardiovascular disease: A systematic review and meta-analysis. Journal of the American Medical Association. 2008;**300**(21):2514-2526. DOI: 10.1001/jama.2008.758

[23] Aboudalle I, Kantarjian HM, Burger JA, Estrov Z, Ohanian M, Jabbour EJ, et al. Efficacy and safety of generic Imatinib after switching from innovator Imatinib in patients treated for chronic myeloid Leukemia. Blood. 2017;**130**:2906. Retrieved from: http://www.bloodjournal.org/content/130/Suppl_1/2906

[24] Howland RH. Are generic medications safe and effective? Journal of Psychosocial Nursing and Mental Health Services. 2010;**48**(3):13-16. DOI: 10.3928/02793695-20100204-01

[25] Sacha T, Góra-Tybor J, Szarejko M, Bober G, Grzybowska-Izydorczyk O, Niesiobędzka-Krężel J, et al. A multicenter prospective study on efficacy and safety of imatinib generics: A report from polish adult Leukemia group imatinib generics registry. American Journal of Hematology.

2017;**92**(7):E125-E128. DOI: 10.1002/ajh.24748

[26] Iyer G, Marimuthu SP, Segal JB, Singh S. An algorithm to identify generic drugs in the FDA adverse event reporting system. Drug Safety. 2017;**40**(9):799-808. DOI: 10.1007/s40264-017-0550-1

[27] Colgan S, Faasse K, Martin LR, Stephens MH, Grey A, Petrie KJ. Perceptions of generic medication in the general population, doctors and pharmacists: A systematic review. British Medical Journal Open. 2015;**5**(12):e008915. DOI: 10.1136/bmjopen-2015-008915

[28] Simoens S. Biosimilar medicines and cost-effectiveness. Clinicoecon Outcomes Reserch. 2011;**3**:29-36. DOI: 10.2147/CEOR.S12494

[29] de Vries TPGM, Henning RH, Hogerzeil HV and Fresle DA: WHO Guide to Good Prescribing—A Practical Manual. Geneva; 1994. Available from: http://apps.who.int/medicinedocs/pdf/whozip23e/whozip23e.pdf [Accessed: 26 January 2019]

[30] Henry D, Taylor C. Pharmacoeconomics of cancer therapies: Considerations with the introduction of biosimilars. Seminars in Oncology. 2014;**41**(Suppl 3):S13-S20. DOI: 10.1053/j.seminoncol.2014.03.009

[31] Garg A, Akku S, Khandarkar S. Cost-minimization analysis of generic equivalents (bortezomib, decitabine and capecitabine) in comparison to the originator brand medicines in Colombia. Generics and Biosimilars Initiative Journal. 2016;**5**(4):164-167. DOI: 10.5639/gabij.2016.0504.042

[32] Pramod K, Tahir MA, Charoo NA, Ansari SH, Ali J. Pharmaceutical product development: A quality by design approach. International Journal of Pharmaceutical Investigation. 2016;**6**(3):129-138. DOI: 10.4103/2230-973X.187350

[33] FDA. Guidance for Industry ANDAs: Stability Testing of Drug Substances and Products. 2014. Available from: https://www.fda.gov/downloads/Drugs/GuidanceComplianceRegulatoryInformation/Guidances/UCM366082.pdf [Accessed: 26 January 2019]

[34] WHO good manufacturing practices for pharmaceutical products: Main principles. 2014. Available from: https://www.who.int/medicines/areas/quality_safety/quality_assurance/production/en/ [Accessed: 26 January 2019]

[35] Schafheutle EI, Hassell K, Noyce PR, Weiss MC. Access to medicines: Cost as an influence on the views and behaviour of patients. Health & Social Care in the Community. 2002;**10**(3):187-195

[36] Allan GM, Lexchin J, Wiebe N. Physician awareness of drug cost: A systematic review. PLoS Medicine. 2007;**4**(9):e283

[37] Mishuk AU, Qian J, Howard JN, Harris I, Frank G, Kiptanui Z, et al. The association between patient sociodemographic characteristics and generic drug use: A systematic review and meta-analysis. Journal of Managed Care Pharmacy. 2018;**24**(3):252-264. DOI: 10.18553/jmcp.2018.24.3.252.

[38] Chu C, Lal LS, Felder TM, Rosenau P. Evaluation of patient assistance program eligibility and availability for top 200 brand name and generic drugs in the United States. Innovations in Pharmacy. 2012;**3**(1):1-9

[39] Bigdeli M, Jacobs B, Tomson G, Laing R, Ghaffar A, Dujardin B, et al. Access to medicines from a health system perspective. Health Policy and Planning. 2013;**28**:692-704. DOI: 10.1093/heapol/czs108

[40] Aivalli PK, Elias MA, Pati MK, Bhanuprakash S, Munegowda C, Shroff

ZC, et al. Perceptions of the quality of generic medicines: Implications for trust in public services within the local health system in Tumkur, India. British Medical Journal Global Health. 2018;**2**:e000644. DOI: 10.1136/bmjgh-2017-000644

[41] Schutte T, Tichelaar J, Nanayakkara P, Richir M, van Agtmael M. Students and doctors are unaware of the cost of drugs they frequently prescribe. Basic & Clinical Pharmacology & Toxicology. 2017;**120**(3):278-283. DOI: 10.1111/bcpt.12678

[42] Flood D, Mathieu I, Chary A, García P, Rohloff P. Perceptions and utilization of generic medicines in Guatemala: A mixed-methods study with physicians and pharmacy staff. BMC Health Services Research. 2017;**17**(1):27

[43] Garg A, Singh AR, Kadukkatt S, Khandarkar S. Perceptions and attitude towards the use of generic drugs by oncologists from emerging markets: A multinational cross sectional survey. International Journal of Scientific Research. 2018;7(12):36-39. DOI: 10.15373/22778179

Chapter 9

Effect of Hyperbaric Oxygen on Hematopoietic Stem Cell Transplantation

Omar S. Aljitawi

Abstract

In this chapter the accumulated evidence that supports the role of hyperbaric oxygen therapy (HBOT) in improving the process of hematopoietic stem/progenitor cell (HSPC) homing, engraftment, and immune-reconstitution will be reviewed. The underlying mechanism by which HBO modulates erythropoietin (EPO)/EPOR signaling to improve HSPC homing and engraftment will be described. Also the pre-clinical evidence and pilot clinical trial evidence that supports HBO role in improving HSPC homing and engraftment will be examined. Current and future clinical trial studies that stem from this concept will be detailed. Finally, areas that need future investigations to optimally utilize HBO in the field of HSPC transplantation will be described.

Keywords: hyperbaric oxygen therapy (HBOT), hematopoietic stem/progenitor cell (HSPC), homing and engraftment, hematopoietic stem/progenitor cell transplantation, pilot clinical trials, phase II clinical trials

1. Introduction

Allogeneic transplantation is the only curative approach for many hematologic malignant and nonmalignant disorders. Unfortunately, only 30% of patients will have a matched sibling donor [1]. However, well-matched donors (MUDs) are a suitable alternative for those who do not. In one study, well-matched MUDs were identified in 53% of those with Northern European ancestry, compared to only 21% of patients of other origin [2]. For patients without a histocompatible adult donor, transplant options include unrelated umbilical cord blood (UCB) transplantation or transplant from a haploidentical (haplo) donor [3]. Since the first successful UCB transplant in 1988 [4], UCB has been used as a graft source for over 40,000 patients with both malignant and nonmalignant diseases [5, 6].

As a graft source for transplantation, UCB has several practical advantages including ease of procurement, absence of donor risks, reduced risk of transmissible infections, and availability for immediate use [7]. UCB is also associated with a lower incidence of graft-versus-host disease (GVHD) despite HLA disparity [8]. Therefore, UCB extends the application of allogeneic transplant to ethnic minority populations who are underrepresented in donor registries [9]. Additionally, UCB transplantation is associated with reduced leukemia relapse in patients with evidence of minimal residual disease at time of transplant, suggesting a strong graft-versus-leukemia effect [10]. However, UCB units in themselves are limited in

IntechOpen

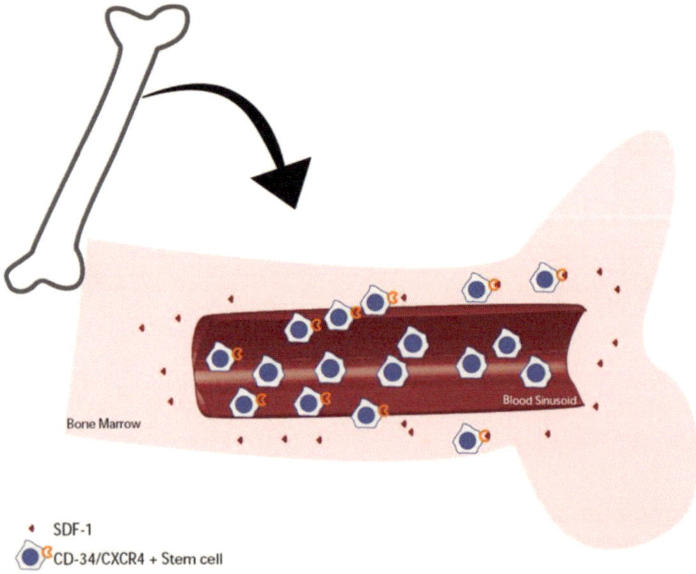

Figure 1.
Hematopoietic stem/progenitor cell (HSPC) homing to the bone marrow. This process is mediated by CXCR4 receptors on the surface of HSPCs and stromal cell-derived factor-1 (SDF-1) in the bone marrow.

cell doses available for optimal transplantation in adults. UCB stem cells also demonstrate defects in homing to the bone marrow (BM), implicating delayed recovery of neutrophil and platelet count and achieved engraftment, resulting in higher rates of graft failure [11]. This prolonged time to engraftment is also associated with delayed immune reconstitution after UCB transplantation [12–14], resulting in higher posttransplant infection rates [15]. Strategies to overcome these defects in homing and engraftment are clearly needed in order to make this potentially curative therapy more effective for patients. Additionally, such strategies might apply to other types of hematopoietic stem cell (HSC) transplantation, including autologous stem cell transplantation as well as allogeneic stem cell transplantation.

Homing is the first process by which circulating hematopoietic cells actively cross the blood/BM endothelium barrier to migrate into the BM compartment (**Figure 1**) [16]. This process is fairly rapid and occurs within hours and no longer than a day or two after stem cell infusion [16]. HSC homing is mediated in part by the binding of chemokine CXCR4 receptor on the surface of HSCs to their ligand, stromal cell-derived factor-1 (SDF-1) expressed by BM stromal cells [17]. Stem cell homing precedes engraftment, corresponding to proliferation and differentiation of hematopoietic stem cells (HSCs) to produce mature, functional hematopoietic cells within the BM [18]. One study claimed that only 18–20% of all intravenously transplanted stem cells, including different subsets, seeded in the BM, with UCB stem cell seeding even lower [19]. Another study demonstrated that human UCB stem cell seeding efficiency in NOD/SCID mice was found to be less than that for BM (4.4% versus 20%) [20].

2. Current methods to improve UCB HSPC homing

Due to the curative potential of UCB transplantation, several approaches have been investigated to improve UCB stem cell homing to the BM. In one study inhibition of CD26 peptidase activity by pretreating purified $CD34^+$ human CB cells with

Diprotin A significantly enhanced engraftment of HSCs from human UCB into NOD/SCID mice [21]. A CD26 peptidase inhibitor, sitagliptin, was investigated in a clinical trial with encouraging results in engraftment of adults with hematological malignancies after using a single unit UCB transplant [22]. Another strategy taken involved direct intrabone administration of cord blood cells into the superior-posterior iliac crest under rapid general anesthesia. Though this strategy produced impressive results in one study [23], another study showed contradictory results [24]. Therefore this procedure has not been widely accepted. In exploring further defects in cord blood stem cell homing, it was found that cord blood $CD34^+$ cells have reduced alpha(1,3)-fucosyltransferase (FucT) expression and activity causing a depletion of cord blood stem cell surface ligands necessary for interaction with adhesion molecules at time of stem cell homing [25]. Forcing fucosylation was found to be clinically feasible with encouraging engraftment efficiency data in the double UCB transplant setting [26]. Some of these interventions require significant logistical support, and some require graft manipulation; accordingly, there is an urgent need to identify safe and practical interventions to enhance UCB homing and engraftment for patients with hematologic malignancies who are undergoing allogeneic stem cell transplantation.

3. Pre-clinical data supporting HBO role in modulating EPO/EPOR signaling in HSCs

Previously published work implicating erythropoietin (EPO) in HSC homing led investigators to examine the role of EPO/EPOR signaling in HSC homing and engraftment in vitro and in vivo pre-clinical models. Gonzalez et al. demonstrated that circulating HSCs rapidly decline after birth [27]. Interestingly, the decline in HSCs correlated with low EPO blood concentration. Additionally, the decline in HSCs being attributed to HSC BM homing, these observations suggested a possible role for EPO in BM homing and clearance of HSCs from the infant's circulation following birth. Investigators have pursued HBO as a potentially safe approach to effectively lower EPO as previously published [28]. The hypothesis was that lowering EPO at the time of hematopoietic stem/progenitor cell (HSPC) infusion will result in improved bone marrow homing and subsequent engraftment. Studies examining HBOT effects on hematopoietic stem cells are limited. On the other hand, HBOT has been shown to have minimal, if any, effects on blood counts during steady-state conditions [29]. The previously published and accumulated pre-clinical data that supports EPO's role in UCB engraftment are summarized in the next section [30].

To understand EPO effects on UCB $CD34^+$, the expression of EPOR was assessed by flow cytometry. Analyses of 5 UCB units revealed that on average 6.5% of $CD34^+$ UCB cells express EPOR [30]. A significantly higher percentage of EPOR positive cells (45.7 ± 1.4%, **Figure 2**) was observed within the HSC (Lin^- $CD34^+$ $CD38^-$ $CD45RA^-$ $CD90^+$ $CD49f^+$ cells) population. EPOR positive cells were less among multipotent progenitor (MPP) (Lin^- $CD34^+$ $CD38^-$ $CD45RA^-$ $CD90^-$ $CD49f^-$ cells, 22.2 ± 0.3%) or the broader progenitor pool ($Lin^-CD34^+CD38^+$ cells, 25.1 ± 0.7%). To test whether a functional EPO-EPOR signaling cascade was activated in EPOR-expressing UCB $CD34^+$ cells, EPOR expression was depleted via RNA interference (RNAi), and the erythroid differentiation potential after culture in methylcellulose culture medium was compared to UCB $CD34^+$ cells without EPOR depletion. Depletion of EPOR expression by RNAi greatly reduced the size of erythroid colonies and UCB $CD34^+$ differentiation potential toward the erythroid lineage, indicating that EPO promotes functional EPO-EPOR signaling response in these cells [30].

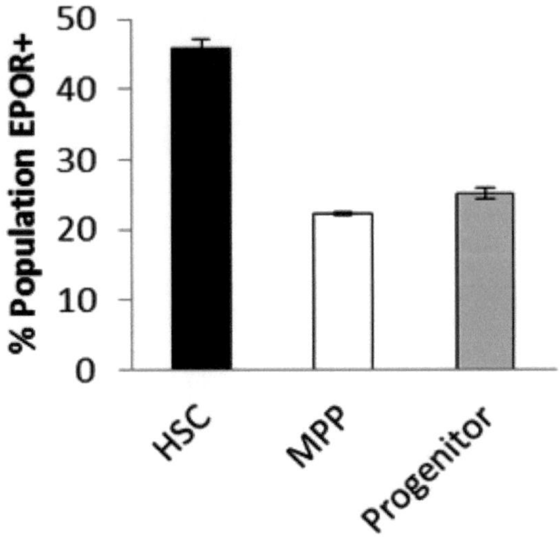

Figure 2.
Erythropoietin receptor expression on umbilical cord blood CD34⁺ cells and subsets (unpublished data).

As earlier studies potentially implicated EPO signaling in hematopoietic stem/progenitor cell (HSPC) homing [27], investigators tested if there were EPO-EPOR signaling effects on SDF-1-induced migration of UCB $CD34^+$ HSPC, by examining UCB $CD34^+$ $CD38^-$ cell transmigration toward an SDF-1 gradient after a preexposure of the cells to different concentrations of EPO. Exposure of UCB $CD34^+$ $CD38^-$ to EPO significantly reduced their SDF-1-induced directional migration. Blocking EPO signaling by anti-EPOR or anti-EPO antibodies rescued SDF-1-induced migration of UCB $CD34^+$ cells for both $CD34^+$ $CD38^-$ and $CD34^+$ $CD38^+$ populations [30].

HBO treatment has been shown to reduce systemic EPO levels in healthy volunteers [28]. As previous in vitro studies indicated that EPO-EPOR signaling inhibits SDF-1-induced migration of UCB $CD34^+$ cells, investigators examined whether HBO pre-treatment of mice prior to cell infusion enhances BM homing. First, investigators measured serum EPO levels in their murine transplant model 7 hours after HBO exposure (or 3 hours post UCB $CD34^+$ infusion). HBO exposure significantly reduced serum EPO levels compared to controls ($p < 0.0001$). In addition, a higher percentage of the UCB $CD34^+$ cells was seen in the BM of HBO-treated mice 3 hours posttransplant [30].

In the same murine model, investigators evaluated the impact of HBO treatment on peripheral blood, BM, and spleen retention at early time points (24–72 hours), which correlates with BM homing, and up to 4.5 months, which correlates with long-term engraftment. Efficient support of human cell engraftment has been reported in 6–8-week-old female NSG mice NOD/SCID/IL-$2Rgc^{null}$ [31] model. Briefly, sublethally irradiated NSG mice, after 24 hours, were treated with HBO for 2 hours (HBO) or without HBO in the control group. Next, approximately 10^5 CD34-selected UCB cells were infused into each mouse 6 hours following the start of HBO. Mice were euthanized at different time points; peripheral blood, BM, and spleen tissue were harvested; and engraftment was analyzed by flow cytometry. The degree of engraftment was determined by measuring the percentage of human CD45-expressing cells. For HBO therapy, 100% oxygen was delivered at 2.5 atmospheres absolute (ATA) in a single-place chamber. In murine in vivo model, HBO-treated mice had significantly improved BM ($p = 0.0067$), peripheral blood ($p = 0.0131$), and spleen ($p = 0.0293$) engraftment [32], the impact of which was more pronounced toward later time points at 3 and 4 months.

DOI: http://dx.doi.org/10.5772/intechopen.85223

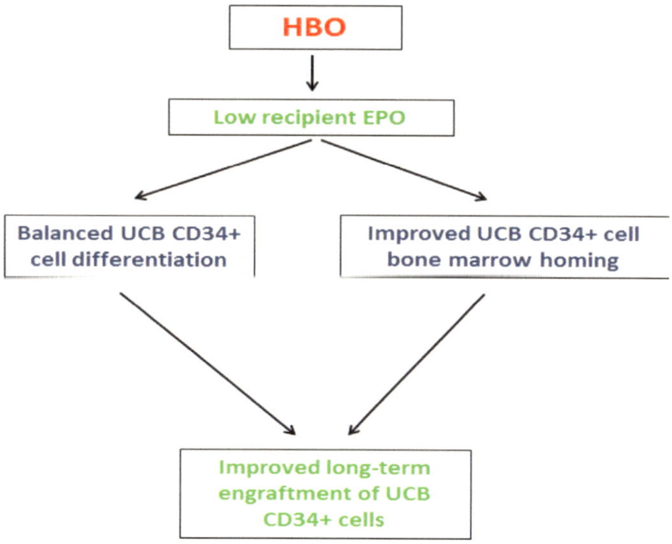

Figure 3.
The mechanisms by which hyperbaric oxygen therapy (HBO) affects hematopoietic stem/progenitor cell engraftment.

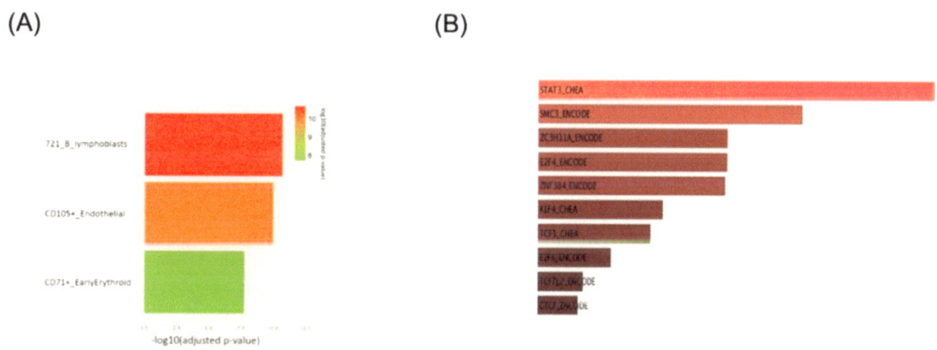

Figure 4.
Gene expression data analysis evaluating erythropoietin (EPO) treatment effects on UCB CD34$^+$ cells. EPO treatment enriches CD71$^+$ early erythroid cells (A) and correlates with active STAT3 signaling (B) (unpublished data).

EPO has been shown to impact hematopoietic progenitor cells differentiation [33]. Because HBOT lowers EPO levels in posttransplant, the impact of a low EPO environment induced by HBO on human UCB CD34$^+$ cell differentiation was examined. HBO mice demonstrated significantly lower numbers of burst-forming unit-erythroid (BFU-E) ($p = 0.043$) and increasing numbers of colony-forming unit-granulocyte/macrophage (CFU-G/M) ($p = 0.05$) 1 week following transplant. Interestingly, despite reduced BFU-E in the in vivo experiments, investigators observed a favorable trend in red blood cell (RBC) time to transfusion independence (TTI) in their pilot study.

These findings suggest that lowering the recipient EPO levels favors UCB CD34$^+$ engraftment by affecting two important HSC functions: BM homing and HSPC differentiation (**Figure 3**). Lower recipient EPO at the time of UCB CD34$^+$ cell infusion results in less early erythroid differentiation of infused progenitor cells. This leads to early homing of undifferentiated UCB CD34$^+$ cells to the BM, thus improving long-term multi-lineage engraftment. In confirmatory experiments utilizing

RNA-seq for transcriptional assessment, investigators found that EPO treatment of UCB $CD34^+$ cells enriches $CD71^+$ early erythroid cells, consistent with early erythroid commitment (**Figure 4**). In the same data set, EPO treatment was associated with signal transducer and activator of transcription 3 (STAT3) pathway activation (**Figure 4**). Importantly, signal transducer and activator of transcription 3 (STAT3) is a known downstream effector of EPOR signal transduction [34–37].

4. Pilot clinical data supporting HBO role in HSC transplantation

To date, two pilot clinical trials exploring HBO in UCB transplantation as well as autologous hematopoietic cell transplantation (HCT) have been completed. In both studies HBO was given in standard fashion at least 6 hours prior to HSCP infusion on day 0 of their transplant (**Figure 5**). The first aim of these studies is to examine the safety and tolerability of HBO in the setting of HCT. In addition, these studies explored the impact of HBO on blood count recovery as well as EPO levels posttransplant. Details of HBO therapy and the results of these studies are being summarized in the next three paragraphs.

4.1 Details of HBO therapy

After receiving routine clinical care on day 0 (the day of HSPC infusion), subjects were exposed to HBO for a total of 90 min after compression to 2.5 atmosphere absolutes (ATA) in a monoplace hyperbaric chamber (Model 3200/3200R, Sechrist Industries, Inc., USA), breathing 100% oxygen. The subjects spent 10–15 min during the compression and decompression phases and 10 min room air breaks for every 30 min of HBO treatment.

4.2 HBO in UCB transplantation

Based on the previously mentioned pre-clinical data, a pilot clinical trial investigating the safety of HBO in UCB transplant was initiated. Patients considered

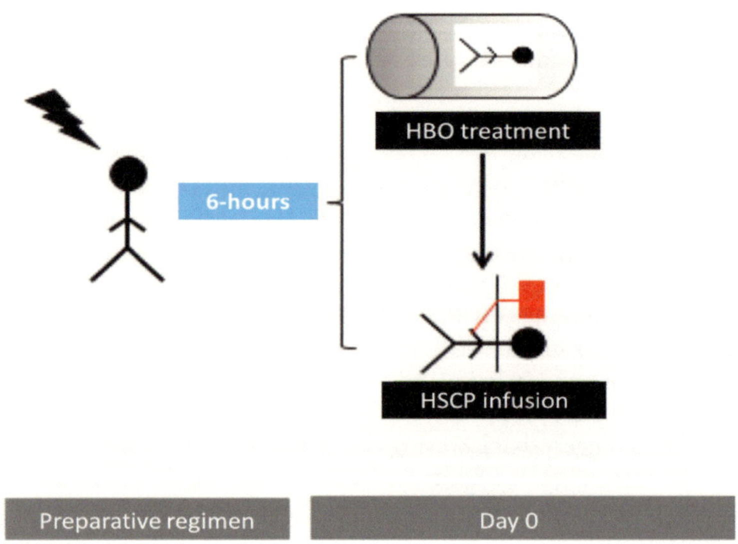

Figure 5.
Clinical trial schema incorporating hyperbaric oxygen (HBO) into hematopoietic cell transplantation.

		HBO (n = 15)	Historic (n = 48)	p value
Neutrophil recovery (n/%)	No	0%	6 (12%)	NS
	Yes	15 (100%)	42 (82%)	
Platelet recovery (n/%)	No	0%	15 (31%)	0.013
	Yes	15 (100%)	33 (69%)	
Median time to neutrophil recovery (range)		14 (6–45)	20.5 (571)	NS
Median time to platelet recovery (range)		37.5 (0–85)	38 (0–161)	NS

Table 1.
Blood count recovery in umbilical cord blood transplantation pilot study utilizing hyperbaric oxygen (HBO).

for either standard myeloablative conditioning (MAC) (higher intensity chemotherapy and radiation) or standard reduced intensity conditioning (RIC) (lesser intensity chemotherapy and radiation) UCB transplantation were enrolled. In this study, HBO treatment was administered on day 0 of the transplant. The treatment consisted of exposure to 100% oxygen at 2.5 ATA for a total of 2 hours, in a single see-through hyperbaric chamber. Six hours from the start of HBO, single or double UCB units are infused, and patients are followed daily for toxicity and blood count recovery. In addition to safety, neutrophil and platelet recovery and engraftment were investigated as efficacy end points. A total of 15 subjects have been treated; all have tolerated the procedure very well except for 1 patient who did not finish the last 10 min of therapy because of nausea thought to be secondary to a concomitant medication. In terms of efficacy, final data from the study indicate an encouraging median time to neutrophil recovery of 14 days compared to 20.5 in historic data (n = 48) and a median time to platelet count recovery of 37.5 compared to 38 in historic data (**Table 1**). HBO also resulted in improved day 100 survival (p = 0.051) and in improvement in the percentage of patients who demonstrated Neutrophil recovery was not significant platelet count recovery (p = 0.013). HBO also resulted in statistically significant reduction in median EPO level from baseline (−30.37 mU/ml+/−31.68, p = 0.004).

In a follow-up study, the long-term outcome of patients in this pilot HBO study in UCB transplantation was examined. Patients' outcome was compared to a historic control group. The 6-month survival in the HBO group was 100%, compared to 67.0% in the control group (95% CI 50.1–79.4%, $p < 0.0001$) [38]. HBO-treated patients had on average lower relapse and non-relapse mortality rates, and less chronic graft-versus-host disease (GVHD), but had increased acute GVHD. However, these differences were not statistically significant, probably because of the small sample size. In the HBO-treated cohort, immune-reconstitution analysis showed significant improvement in early B-cell recovery, with a trend toward improvement in early NK cell recovery. The ratio of 8 hours to baseline EPO levels was examined. A nonsignificant trend toward lower EPO values was found in those who did not relapse or die in year 1 than those who did die or relapse. Disease progression-free survival was also improved in those who had more than 80% reduction in EPO levels in response to HBO. This study highlights the long-term safety of HBO therapy when used prior to UCB transplantation. It also shows a relationship between HBO-induced EPO reduction, early NK cell recovery and posttransplant disease progression. Since lower rates of relapse have been reported in association with higher early NK cell recovery [39], it was hypothesized that by reducing EPO, HBO improves early NK cell recovery, and improved NK cell recovery slows down disease progression.

4.3 HBO in autologous HCT

Encouraged by the results of HBO in UCB transplantation, the same group conducted a pilot study in Auto-HSPC transplantation. A total of 20 patients were treated on the Auto-HSPC transplant study. HBO therapy was very well tolerated as 19 completed full therapy [40]. For efficacy comparison, HBO subjects were matched to historical controls from the same institution based on gender, age (within 5 years), disease type (multiple myeloma or lymphoma), and preparative regimen. The median time to neutrophil count recovery was 11 days in both cohorts, the HBO and control cohorts. However, time to neutrophil recovery was approximately 1 day sooner for HBO than historical controls taking into account the full distribution estimates of Kaplan-Meier estimator (log rank $p = 0.005$). The median time to platelet count recovery was 16 versus 18 days for the HBO and control cohorts, respectively (log rank $p < 0.0001$).

In a separate analysis, HBO effects on other outcomes of post-autologous transplantation were evaluated. In this analysis, the HBO cohort patients who completed HBO therapy ($n = 19$) were compared with historic patients ($n = 225$) [40]. The average days of GCSF use were 6 days in the HBO cohort compared to 8 days in controls ($p < 0.01$). Also, HBO patients had significantly less mucositis (26.3 versus 64.2%, $p < 0.01$).

5. HBO and stem cell mobilization

In the previous section, the effects of HBO on stem cell homing and engraftment posttransplant were reviewed. Interestingly, HBO can also help with stem cell/progenitor cell mobilization from the bone marrow [41]. However, the mobilized stem/progenitor cells exhibited characteristics of endothelial progenitor cells [42].

6. Current and future prospective

Incorporating HBO into HCT backbone represents a new direction in the field of HCT aiming at improving the outcome of HCT by improving HSPC homing and subsequent engraftment. Accumulated data suggest improvement in immune reconstitution too. Targeting EPO at the time of HSPC infusion represents a new understanding of EPO role in basic HSCP functions, including cell differentiation, transmigration, homing, and engraftment. Though these studies represent an early attempt at understanding EPO role in HSCP biologic functions and HBO's role in blocking EPO/EPOR signaling in HCT transplantation, the accumulated data seem to be promising. Currently, a phase II study investigating HBO in Auto-HCT is open for enrollment (ClinicalTrials.gov Identifier: NCT03398200). Another phase II study investigating HBO in UCB transplantation is expected to be open for enrollment in early 2019 (ClinicalTrials.gov Identifier: NCT03739502). Both of these studies are randomized prospective clinical trials that focus on investigating HBO effects on time to neutrophil recovery, platelet count recovery, blood and platelet transfusion requirements, and growth factor use. Additionally, both studies will be evaluating disease response posttransplant. Immune reconstitution will be examined in an attempt to correlate that to disease response posttransplant, hypothesizing that HBOT improves immune reconstitution which in turn will result in improved disease response to transplant. Finally, these studies will examine HBO effects on EPO and IL-15 levels posttransplant. The study in UCB transplantation will also focus on time to achieving full-donor chimerism as that might influence disease control posttransplant. This wave of phase II studies will be essential in establishing the efficacy of such procedure in HCT and might lead to future phase III studies.

An additional area for future investigation is defining the optimal HBO schedule to effectively block EPO/EPOR signaling during HCT. In a previous study, one single HBO treatment 6 hours prior to HSPC infusion was used. It was noticed that EPO level rebounds as early as 24 hours after HBO treatment [30]; accordingly additional HBO therapy might keep EPO levels low for 48 hours, which is the duration during which homing occurs. To accomplish that, investigators will have to treat the recipients 24 hours after HSPC infusion, which means the infused HSPCs will be exposed to hyperbaric conditions. In their experience, direct $CD34^+$ cell exposure to HBO reduced their proliferation, impaired their in vitro transmigration, and reduced their erythroid differentiation [43]. These effects were statistically significant, but the biological effects were minimal which in theory should not influence UCB $CD34^+$ cell behavior significantly. Additionally, these direct HBO effects on UCB $CD34^+$ cells are desirable when it comes to the HSPCs that have already homed to the bone marrow as these effects might help with HSPC retention in the bone marrow.

Finally, in addition to reducing EPO and affecting EPO/EPOR signaling, HBO might have additional effects beyond EPO/EPOR signaling that might impact HSPC biologic functions.

7. Conclusions

Targeting EPO using HBO in hematopoietic cell transplantation is a new direction in the HCT field which will potentially have major impact on the outcome of HCT. By improving HSPC homing, engraftment, and immune reconstitution, HBO therapy will have the potential to improve the outcome of HCT by improving patient recovery and by reducing posttransplant complications related to infections. Overall, that might reduce the cost of HCT. Though data from pre-clinical and pilot clinical studies are encouraging, data from current and future phase II studies might show more definitive data in support of this application. Also future studies will be needed to examine HBO effects on bone marrow microenvironment elements.

Conflict of interest

No conflict of interest to declare.

Author details

Omar S. Aljitawi
University of Rochester Medical Center, Rochester, NY, USA

*Address all correspondence to: omar_aljitawi@urmc.rochester.edu

References

[1] Barker JN, Wagner JE. Umbilical-cord blood transplantation for the treatment of cancer. Nature Reviews. Cancer. 2003;**3**(7):526-532

[2] Barker JN, Byam CE, Kernan NA, Lee SS, Hawke RM, Doshi KA, et al. Availability of cord blood extends allogeneic hematopoietic stem cell transplant access to racial and ethnic minorities. Biology of Blood and Marrow Transplantation: Journal of the American Society for Blood and Marrow Transplantation. 2010;**16**(11):1541-1548

[3] Ruggeri A, Ciceri F, Gluckman E, Labopin M, Rocha V. Alternative donors hematopoietic stem cells transplantation for adults with acute myeloid leukemia: Umbilical cord blood or haploidentical donors? Best Practice & Research. Clinical Haematology. 2010;**23**(2):207-216

[4] Gluckman E, Broxmeyer HA, Auerbach AD, Friedman HS, Douglas GW, Devergie A, et al. Hematopoietic reconstitution in a patient with Fanconi's anemia by means of umbilical-cord blood from an HLA-identical sibling. The New England Journal of Medicine. 1989;**321**(17):1174-1178

[5] Ballen KK, Gluckman E, Broxmeyer HE. Umbilical cord blood transplantation: The first 25 years and beyond. Blood. 25 Jul 2013;**122**(4): 491-498. DOI: 10.1182/blood-2013-02-453175. [Epub: 14 May 2013]

[6] Ruggeri A. Alternative donors: Cord blood for adults. Seminars in Hematology. 2016;**53**(2):65-73

[7] Gluckman E. History of cord blood transplantation. Bone Marrow Transplantation. 2009;**44**(10):621-626

[8] Laughlin MJ. Umbilical cord blood for allogeneic transplantation in children and adults. Bone Marrow Transplantation. 2001;**27**(1):1-6

[9] Johansen KA, Schneider JF, McCaffree MA, Woods GL. Efforts of the United States' National Marrow Donor Program and registry to improve utilization and representation of minority donors. Transfusion Medicine. 2008;**18**(4):250-259

[10] Milano F, Gooley T, Wood B, Woolfrey A, Flowers ME, Doney K, et al. Cord-blood transplantation in patients with minimal residual disease. The New England Journal of Medicine. 2016;**375**(10):944-953

[11] Migliaccio AR, Adamson JW, Stevens CE, Dobrila NL, Carrier CM, Rubinstein P. Cell dose and speed of engraftment in placental/umbilical cord blood transplantation: Graft progenitor cell content is a better predictor than nucleated cell quantity. Blood. 2000;**96**(8):2717-2722

[12] Szabolcs P, Niedzwiecki D. Immune reconstitution after unrelated cord blood transplantation. Cytotherapy. 2007;**9**(2):111-122

[13] Brown JA, Boussiotis VA. Umbilical cord blood transplantation: Basic biology and clinical challenges to immune reconstitution. Clinical Immunology. 2008;**127**(3):286-297

[14] Komanduri KV, St John LS, de Lima M, McMannis J, Rosinski S, McNiece I, et al. Delayed immune reconstitution after cord blood transplantation is characterized by impaired thymopoiesis and late memory T-cell skewing. Blood. 2007;**110**(13):4543-4551

[15] Szabolcs P, Cairo MS. Unrelated umbilical cord blood transplantation and immune reconstitution. Seminars in Hematology. 2010;**47**(1):22-36

[16] Lapidot T, Dar A, Kollet O. How do stem cells find their way home? Blood. 2005;**106**(6):1901-1910

[17] Lapidot T, Kollet O. The brain-bone-blood triad: Traffic lights for stem-cell homing and mobilization. Hematology. American Society of Hematology. Education Program. 2010;**2010**:1-6

[18] Nilsson SK, Simmons PJ. Transplantable stem cells: Home to specific niches. Current Opinion in Hematology. 2004;**11**(2):102-106

[19] van der Loo JC, Ploemacher RE. Marrow- and spleen-seeding efficiencies of all murine hematopoietic stem cell subsets are decreased by preincubation with hematopoietic growth factors. Blood. 1995;**85**(9):2598-2606

[20] Yahata T, Ando K, Sato T, Miyatake H, Nakamura Y, Muguruma Y, et al. A highly sensitive strategy for SCID-repopulating cell assay by direct injection of primitive human hematopoietic cells into NOD/SCID mice bone marrow. Blood. 2003;**101**(8):2905-2913

[21] Campbell TB, Hangoc G, Liu Y, Pollok K, Broxmeyer HE. Inhibition of CD26 in human cord blood CD34$^+$ cells enhances their engraftment of nonobese diabetic/severe combined immunodeficiency mice. Stem Cells and Development. 2007;**16**(3):347-354

[22] Farag SS, Srivastava S, Messina-Graham S, Schwartz J, Robertson MJ, Abonour R, et al. *In vivo* DPP-4 inhibition to enhance engraftment of single-unit cord blood transplants in adults with hematological malignancies. Stem Cells and Development. 2013;**22**(7):1007-1015

[23] Frassoni F, Gualandi F, Podesta M, Raiola AM, Ibatici A, Piaggio G, et al. Direct intrabone transplant of unrelated cord-blood cells in acute leukaemia: A phase I/II study. The Lancet Oncology. 2008;**9**(9):831-839

[24] Brunstein CG, Barker JN, Weisdorf DJ, Defor TE, McKenna D, Chong SY, et al. Intra-BM injection to enhance engraftment after myeloablative umbilical cord blood transplantation with two partially HLA-matched units. Bone Marrow Transplantation. 2009;**43**(12):935-940

[25] Hidalgo A, Frenette PS. Enforced fucosylation of neonatal CD34$^+$ cells generates selectin ligands that enhance the initial interactions with microvessels but not homing to bone marrow. Blood. 2005;**105**(2):567-575

[26] Popat U, Mehta RS, Rezvani K, Fox P, Kondo K, Marin D, et al. Enforced fucosylation of cord blood hematopoietic cells accelerates neutrophil and platelet engraftment after transplantation. Blood. 2015;**125**(19):2885-2892

[27] Gonzalez S, Amat L, Azqueta C, Madrigal JA, Lailla JM, Garcia J, et al. Factors modulating circulation of hematopoietic progenitor cells in cord blood and neonates. Cytotherapy. 2009;**11**(1):35-42

[28] Balestra C, Germonpre P, Poortmans JR, Marroni A. Serum erythropoietin levels in healthy humans after a short period of normobaric and hyperbaric oxygen breathing: The "normobaric oxygen paradox". Journal of Applied Physiology. 2006;**100**(2):512-518

[29] Gunes AE, Aktas S. Effect of hyperbaric oxygen therapy on complete blood count. Undersea & Hyperbaric Medicine. 2017;**44**(4):357-364

[30] Aljitawi OS, Paul S, Ganguly A, Lin TL, Ganguly S, Vielhauer G, et al. Erythropoietin modulation is associated with improved homing and engraftment post umbilical cord blood transplantation. Blood. 22 Dec 2016;**128**(25):3000-3010. DOI: 10.1182/blood-2016-05-715292. [Epub: 2016 Oct 19]

[31] Ito M, Hiramatsu H, Kobayashi K, Suzue K, Kawahata M, Hioki K, et al. NOD/SCID/gamma(c)(null) mouse: An excellent recipient mouse model for engraftment of human cells. Blood. 2002;**100**(9):3175-3182

[32] Aljitawi OS, Xiao Y, Eskew JD, Parelkar NK, Swink M, Radel J, et al. Hyperbaric oxygen improves engraftment of *ex-vivo* expanded and gene transduced human CD34(+) cells in a murine model of umbilical cord blood transplantation. Blood Cells, Molecules & Diseases. 2014;**52**(1):59-67

[33] Grover A, Mancini E, Moore S, Mead AJ, Atkinson D, Rasmussen KD, et al. Erythropoietin guides multipotent hematopoietic progenitor cells toward an erythroid fate. The Journal of Experimental Medicine. 2014;**211**(2):181-188

[34] Cao Y, Lathia JD, Eyler CE, Wu Q, Li Z, Wang H, et al. Erythropoietin receptor signaling through STAT3 is required for glioma stem cell maintenance. Genes & Cancer. 2010;**1**(1):50-61

[35] Wincewicz A, Sulkowska M, Koda M, Lesniewicz T, Kanczuga-Koda L, Sulkowski S. STAT3, HIF-1alpha, EPO and EPOR—Signaling proteins in human primary ductal breast cancers. Folia Histochemica et Cytobiologica. 2007;**45**(2):81-86

[36] Acs G, Acs P, Beckwith SM, Pitts RL, Clements E, Wong K, et al. Erythropoietin and erythropoietin receptor expression in human cancer. Cancer Research. 2001;**61**(9):3561-3565

[37] Kirito K, Nakajima K, Watanabe T, Uchida M, Tanaka M, Ozawa K, et al. Identification of the human erythropoietin receptor region required for Stat1 and Stat3 activation. Blood. 2002;**99**(1):102-110

[38] Mina A, Shune L, Abdelhakim H, Lin TL, Ganguly S, Baran A, et al. Long-term results of a pilot study evaluating hyperbaric oxygen therapy to improve umbilical cord blood engraftment. Annals of Hematology. Feb 2019;**98**(2):481-489. DOI: 10.1007/s00277-018-3532-1. Epub: 2018 Oct 31

[39] Huttunen P, Taskinen M, Siitonen S, Saarinen-Pihkala UM. Impact of very early CD4(+)/CD8(+) T cell counts on the occurrence of acute graft-versus-host disease and NK cell counts on outcome after pediatric allogeneic hematopoietic stem cell transplantation. Pediatric Blood & Cancer. 2015;**62**(3):522-528

[40] Abdelhakim H, Shune L, Bhatti S, Cantilena AR, Baran A, Lin TL, et al. Results of the first clinical study in humans that combines hyperbaric oxygen pre-treatment with autologous peripheral blood stem cell transplantation. Biology of Blood and Marrow Transplantation: Journal of the American Society for Blood and Marrow Transplantation. 3 Jun 2019. pii: S1083-8791(19)30353-2. DOI: 10.1016/j.bbmt.2019.05.028. [Epub ahead of print]

[41] Thom SR, Bhopale VM, Velazquez OC, Goldstein LJ, Thom LH, Buerk DG. Stem cell mobilization by hyperbaric oxygen. American Journal of Physiology. Heart and Circulatory Physiology. 2006;**290**(4):H1378-H1386

[42] Goldstein LJ, Gallagher KA, Bauer SM, Bauer RJ, Baireddy V, Liu Z-J, et al. Endothelial progenitor cell release into circulation is triggered by hyperoxia-induced increases in bone marrow nitric oxide. Stem Cells. 2006;**24**(10):2309-2318

[43] Cheung KY, Berry A, Li D, Aljitawi OS. Hyperbaric oxygen treatment effects on *in vitro* cultured umbilical cord blood CD34+ cells. Cytotherapy. 2018;**20**(1):87-94